DERMATOLOGY - LABORATORY AND CLINICAL RESEARCH

SKIN AGING AND PHOTOAGING

PHYSIOLOGY, CLINICAL ASPECTS AND EMERGING THERAPIES

DERMATOLOGY - LABORATORY AND CLINICAL RESEARCH

Additional books in this series can be found on Nova's website under the Series tab.

Additional e-books in this series can be found on Nova's website under the e-book tab.

DERMATOLOGY - LABORATORY AND CLINICAL RESEARCH

SKIN AGING AND PHOTOAGING

PHYSIOLOGY, CLINICAL ASPECTS AND EMERGING THERAPIES

EMANUEL GRAHAM
EDITOR

NOVA BIOMEDICAL
New York

Library of Congress Cataloging-in-Publication Data

ISBN: 978-1-63482-907-6
Library of Congress Control Number: 2015939745

Published by Nova Science Publishers, Inc. † New York

Contents

Preface

Skin aging is the result of two distinct, biological processes which may occur concurrently: extrinsic and intrinsic aging. The first chapter of this book focuses on the anti-skin aging effects of natural products, such as polyphenols and terpenes using topical application and oral administration. Future prospects for this field of research will focus on natural products combined with molecular techniques to help maximize the desired anti-skin aging benefits. The second chapter provides a brief review of skin characteristics, skin aging mechanisms and dermal applications. The next chapter of the book reviews the types of pollution and external aggression that skin is exposed to and reviews recently published studies that report that cumulative exposure to the five daily environmental aggressors (pollution, sun, cold, heat and wind) increase this skin damage. The remaining chapters review the role of inflammation in regulation of skin aging; the relevant methods, the physiological structure and function of the Stratum Corneum, as well as the effects of intrinsic and extrinsic aging on these parameters; the physiology of skin photoaging and the emerging therapies for combating photoaging and photocarcingenesis; and the biological effects and the latest findings on the role of macrophage migration inhibitory factors (MIF) in photoaging following UV exposure.

In: Skin Aging and Photoaging
Editor: Emanuel Graham
ISBN: 978-1-63482-907-6

Chapter 1

An Insight into Anti-Skin Aging Effects of Natural Products: Topical Application and Oral Administration

Bin Du[1,2], Fengmei Zhu[1] and Baojun Xu[2,*]
[1]Hebei Normal University of Science and Technology, Qinhuangdao, Hebei, China
[2]Food Science and Technology Program, Beijing Normal University–Hong Kong Baptist University United International College, Zhuhai, Guangdong, China

Abstract

Skin aging is the result of two distinct, biological processes which may occur concurrently: extrinsic aging and intrinsic aging. Extrinsic aging of the skin is exemplified by deep, coarse wrinkles, mottled hyperpigmentation and a marked loss of elasticity and recoil. On the other hand, intrinsically aged skin is a slow process which causes changes in tissue structure and impairs function in the absence of additional

* Author to whom correspondence should be addressed. Full postal address: 28, Jinfeng Road, Tangjiawan, Zhuhai, Guangdong 519085, China. Tel.:+86 756 3620636; fax: +86 756 3620882. E-mail: baojunxu@uic.edu.hk (B.J. Xu).

chemical, biological and physical factors. Our skin provides a very efficient delivery system for chemicals to enter the body. Unfortunately our skin also absorbs toxic chemicals commonly found in personal care products. Consequently, we should switch to natural skin care products. There has been a very long history in human civilization of the usage of natural products; such as herbs, roots, essential oils and flowers for skin care. A cosmetic formulation including natural products can protect the skin against exogenous or endogenous harmful agents, and help to remedy many skin conditions. Although there are several treatments available for aged skin, oral administration supplements and topical application formulations remain the best approach and should be encouraged to all patients. This chapter focuses on the anti-skin aging effects of natural products, such as polyphenols and terpenes using topical application and oral administration. Future prospective for this field of research will focus on natural products combined with molecular techniques; it will help to maximize the desired anti-skin aging benefits.

Abbreviation

Epigallocatechin gallate EGCG
Ultraviolet UV
Panax ginseng C.A. Meyer root extract PGRE
Quercetin QUER
Quercetin caprylate QU-CAP
Green tea polyphenols GTPs
Carboxymethylated beta-1,3-glucan CM-glucan
Reactive oxygen species ROS
Matrix metalloproteinases MMPs
Illicium anisatum extract IAE
Cyclooxygenase-2 COX-2
Coenzyme Q10 Co Q10
Coprisin A3 CopA3

1. Introduction

Skin, of course, is a complex organ covering the entire surface of the body, and it is vital to have good active immune system. Skin changes associated with chronologic aging or photo-aging, such as wrinkling, laxity, and changes in pigmentation, prompt patients to seek cosmetic procedures to improve the appearance of their skin (Khavkin and Ellis, 2011). Histological changes during the photo-aging of skin include hyperproliferation of keratinocytes and melanocytes (Tanaka et al., 2013). Age-related changes and environmental stresses affect all of the cellular elements in the skin. Skin damage is a consequence of the chronological aging process (Varani, 2010). The use of plants is as old as mankind and in the coming years, the market will see many new products containing natural oils and herbs. Natural botanical compounds as a key ingredient in skin care products have received recent attention and validation of efficacy (Baxter, 2008). Herbal 'total extracts' as well as 'selective extracts' are used in cosmetics (Aburjai and Natsheh, 2003). Plants were once the main source and foundation of cosmetics for anti-aging. Aging of the skin is fundamentally related to reductions in the levels of Type I collagen, the principal component of the dermal layer of the skin. It is important to introduce an efficient agent for effective management of skin aging; this agent should have the fewest possible side effects and the greatest wrinkle-reducing effect (Lee et al., 2007). Consumers are always interested in maintaining a youthful appearance, and as the global population's median age increases, this market is increasingly expanding (Mukul et al., 2011). A cosmeceutical is an ingredient with medicinal properties that manifests beneficial topical actions and provides protection against degenerative skin conditions. Cosmeceuticals are topically applied, but they contain ingredients that influence the biological function of the skin (Grace, 2002). A topical application is a medication that is applied to the skin to treat ailments via a large range of classes including creams, foams, gels, lotions, and ointments. Pharmacological doses can be achieved with topical delivery, although solubility, stability, and permeation issues are all concerns. One possible way to circumvent the problem of bioavailability for skin disorders is to apply cosmeceutical topically to the skin. This would allow cosmeceuticals to come into direct contact with the area of interest, without the side effects associated with systemic metabolism (Ndiaye et al., 2011). Topical applications or consumption of some fruits and vegetables or their extracts have been recommended for skin health (Roberts et al., 2009). Oral administration is a route of administration where a substance is taken through the mouth. The advantages include convenient, cheap, no need for sterilization and variety of dose forms.

Nutrition and its reflection on skin has always been an interesting topic for scientists and researchers throughout the centuries worldwide. Natural products have been reported to possess potent anti-oxidant properties and have been widely used in the skin care industry either as topically applied agents or oral supplements in an attempt to prolong youthful skin appearance (Schagen et al., 2012). This chapter discusses the anti-skin aging effects of natural products, such as polyphenols, terpenes, polysaccharides, peptides and proteins, alkaloids, saponins, phytoestrogen, coenzyme Q10 and other natural products using topical application and oral administration.

2. The Aging of Our Skin Can Be Divided into Three Broad Processes

The factors that play roles in the aging process are chronological aging, photo-aging, and stochastic damage.

2.1. Chronological Aging

One of the most frequent dermatologic concerns on skin is aging, it is a complex evitable process of human life and scientific researches are revealing many of the possibilities that cause physiological aging as the time passes (Mukherjee et al., 2011). Chronological aging is due to passage of time. The changes occur partially as the result of cumulative endogenous damage due to the continuous formation of reactive oxygen species (ROS) (Puizina-Ivić, 2008). Despite a strong antioxidant defense system, damage generated by ROS affects cellular constituents such as membranes, enzymes, and DNA (Baumann, 2002). At the same time, skin aging is affected by growth factor modifications and hormone activity that declines with age (Puizina-Ivić, 2008). Clinical manifestations of aged skin are xerosis, laxity, wrinkles, slackness, and the occurrence of benign neoplasms such as seborrheic keratoses and cherry angiomas. There are histological features that accompany these changes (Puizina-Ivić, 2008). Factors that contribute to wrinkling include changes in muscles, the loss of subcutaneous fat tissue, gravitational forces, and the loss of substance of facial bones and cartilage (Puizina-Ivić, 2008). In both chronologic aging and photo-aging, decreased expression of procollagen and increased expression of matrix metalloproteinases (MMPs), a group of matrix-degrading enzymes secreted by epidermal keratinocytes and dermal fibroblasts, are characteristics (Cho et al., 2008).

2.2. Photo-Aging

Premature aging occurred due to some environmental factors on skin produces visible signs such as irregular dryness, dark/light pigmentation, sallowness, severe atrophy, telangiectases, premalignant lesions, laxity, leathery appearance and deep wrinkling. Skin aging is thought to be driven by an increased in-situ production of ROS, which result from both a disturbance of mitochondrial function and a cute stress response to different environment insults including solar radiation (Krutmann et al., 2009). There is also good evidence that intrinsic as well as extrinsic skin aging are associated with a depletion of naturally occurring antioxidants that serve as a defense mechanisms against free radical damage (Sander et al., 2002). The two major environmental influences which induce extrinsic aging are: (i) Chronic exposure to solar ultraviolet (UV) irradiation (termed photo-aging) and (ii) smoking (Langton et al., 2010). The sun is the primary exogenous cause among several internal and environmental factors (Baumann, 2007). In sun-exposed skin, the impact of intrinsic aging is exaggerated by environmental insults, mainly UV irradiation, leading to photo-aging. Recently, a central role for telomere-based signaling can be inferred to elucidate the mechanisms of photo-aging (Kosmadaki and Gilchrest, 2004). The results showed that photo-aging was postulated to disrupt the telomere loop, exposing the tandem repeat sequence TTAGGG of the 30 overhang strand and initiating DNA damage signaling through the p53 tumor suppressor protein. It has been suggested that prevention is the best and most effective way to work against extrinsic skin aging effects (Schagen et al., 2012). The use of botanical supplements has received immense interest in recent years to protect human skin from adverse biological effects of solar UV radiation.

2.3. Stochastic Damage

As stochastic damage is explained, the damage is initiated by random cosmic radiation and triggered by free radicals during cell metabolism, which damages cell lipid compounds, especially membrane structures (Puizina-Ivić, 2008). An oxygen molecule with paired electrons is stable, but one with an unpaired electron is very reactive and it takes electrons from other vital components. As result, cell death or mutations appear on skin (Perricone, 2001; Baumann, 2002).

3. Natural Products against Skin Aging

The research for natural products for skin care and anti-skin aging is on-going world-wide. A review by Lall and Kishore (2014) on the botanical sources used for skin care has been recently summarized in South Africa. Current chapter focuses on anti-skin aging effects of natural compounds or crude extracts from natural products. The action mechanism and the applications of the natural compounds are summarized in Table 1.

Table 1. Topical application and oral administration of natural products against skin-aging

Categories of natural products		Mechanisms	Topical application / Oral administration	References
Flavonoids	Epigallocatechin gallate	Attenuate UV-radiation-induced sunburn severity and alterations in epidermal barrier function	Oral administration	Jeon et al., 2009
	Quercetin	Have rejuvenating effect in already senescent fibroblasts	Topical application	Chondrogianni et al., 2010
	Green tea polyphenols	Inhibit the growth and cause the regression of established experimentally-induced nonmalignant skin papilloma in mice	Oral administration	Wang et al., 1992
	Curcumin	Induce heme oxygenase-1 in normal human skin fibroblasts through redox signaling	-	Lima et al., 2011
	Naringenin and hesperetin	Have protective effect against UV-B-induced skin damage	Topical application	Saija et al., 1998
Stilbenes	Silibinin	Inhibit photocarcinogenesis in mice	Topical application	Mallikarjuna et al., 2004
	Resveratrol	Delay UV-induced skin tumorigenesis and reduce the malignant conversion of benign papillomas to squamous cell carcinoma	Oral administration	Kim et al., 2011

Categories of natural products		Mechanisms	Topical application / Oral administration	References
	Resveratrol	Inhibit UVB-mediated increases in skin edema, inflammation, cyclooxygenase and ornithine decarboxylase induction, and generation of hydrogen peroxide and lipid peroxidation	Topical application	Afaq et al., 2003
Carote-noids	Lutein and zeaxanthin	Protect the skin from damage from both UV and visible radiation	-	Roberts et al., 2009; Dreher and Davenport, 2013
Essential oils	Air-dried *Illicium anisatum* essential oil	Have good anti-elastase effects	-	Kim et al., 2009
	Manuka essential oil	Suppress the UVB-induced increase in skin thickness and wrinkle grading	Topical application	Kwon et al., 2013
Polysac-charides	β-Glucan	Alleviate the extrinsic signs of aging	Topical application	Pillai et al., 2006
	Ganoderma lucidum polysacchari des	Have effect on the gene expression of keratinocytes	-	Xie et al., 2008
	Hericium erinaceum polysacchari des	Enhance skin antioxidant enzymes, matrix metalloproteinases-1, tissue inhibitor of metalloproteinases-1 activities and collagen protein levels	Oral administration	Xu et al., 2010
Peptides and proteins	Phosphatidyl serine	Prevent UV-induced reduction in procollagen expression and inhibited UV-induced matrix metalloproteinases-1 expression	Topical application	Cho et al., 2008

Table 1. (Continued)

Categories of natural products		Mechanisms	Topical application / Oral administration	References
	Coprisin A3 peptide	Prevent UV-induced inhibition of type-I procollagen and induction of matrix metalloproteinases-1	-	Kim et al., 2014
Saponins	Ginseng saponins	Induce human Type I procollagen synthesis	Topical application	Lee et al., 2007
Alkaloids	Berberine	Decrease expression of basal and UV-induced matrix metalloproteinases-1 and increase Type I procollagen expression	-	Kim and Chung, 2008
Phyto-estrogen	Genistein	Reduce cyclobutane pyrimidine dimers formation and increase proliferating cell nuclear antigen expression	Topical application	Moore et al., 2006
	Genistein	Reduce skin roughness and wrinkling and epidermal hyperproliferation	Topical application	Wei et al., 2003
	Wild yam bioidentical progesterone	Promote collagen synthesis and improve skin elasticity and moisture retention levels	Topical application	Barnard, 1994
Coenzyme Q10	Coenzyme Q10	Positively influence the age-affected cellular metabolism and enables to combat signs of aging starting at the cellular level	Topical application	Prahl et al., 2008

Categories of natural products		Mechanisms	Topical application / Oral administration	References
Others	Mangiferin	Inhibit UVB-induced mean length and mean depth of skin wrinkle based on skin replica, epidermal thickening, and damage to collagen fiber	-	Kim et al., 2012
	Trehalose	Reduce UVB-induced corneal damage	Topical application	Emanuele et al., 2014
	Piceatannol	Suppress the UVB-induced generation of ROS in the keratinocytes	-	Maruki-Uchida et al., 2013

3.1. Polyphenols

Polyphenols are a structural class of mainly natural, but also synthetic or semisynthetic, organic chemicals characterized by the presences of large multiples of phenol structural units. The use of polyphenols to inhibit chronic UV radiation exposure-induced skin diseases or skin disorders is gaining attention (Nichols and Katiyar, 2010). Treatment with polyphenols, should be effective to enhance resistance to oxidative stress and prevent/improve skin aging (Masaki, 2010). Afaq and Katiyar (2011) discussed in details the photo-protective effects of green tea polyphenols (GTPs), pomegranate fruit extract, grape seed proanthocyanidins and resveratrol on UV-induced skin inflammation, proliferation, immuno-suppression, DNA damage and dysregulation of important cellular signaling pathways. Jeon et al. (2009) investigated the effect of oral administration of epigallocatechin gallate (EGCG) on the UV-induced skin damage. The results suggested UV-radiation-induced sunburn severity and alterations in epidermal barrier function were also attenuated by the oral supplementation of EGCG. In another study, Chondrogianni et al. (2010) supplemented quercetin (QUER) and its derivative, namely quercetin caprylate (QU-CAP) to already senescent fibroblasts, a rejuvenating effect was observed. These results demonstrated that the existences of QUER and QU-CAP can be effectively used through topical application. Mittal et al. (2003) developed a cream-based EGCG formulation for topical application. Treatment with EGCG in hydrophilic cream resulted in exceptionally high protection against photo-carcinogenesis in a hairless mouse model. They also found that treatment with EGCG resulted in significant inhibition of ultraviolet B (UVB)-induced global DNA hypomethylation pattern. Most of the natural polyphenols are pigments, typically yellow, red or purple, and can absorb UV irradiation. Therefore, when applied topically, they can prevent penetration of the irradiation into the skin (Nichols and Katiyar, 2010). Katiyar et al. (1999) investigated whether topical application of EGCG inhibits UVB-induced infiltration of leukocytes in human skin. In this study, human subjects were UVB irradiated on sun-protected skin to four times their minimal erythema dosage and skin biopsies or keratomes were obtained either 24 h or 48 h later. The results found that topical application of EGCG before UVB exposure to human skin significantly blocked UVB-induced infiltration of leukocytes and reduced myeloperoxidase activity. These *in vivo* studies that have been generated using both animal and human systems provide insights into the possible protective mechanisms involved in the anti-aging effects of polyphenols.

Additionally, Wang et al. (1992) found that oral feeding of GTPs to mice to inhibit the growth and/or caused the regression of established experimentally-induced nonmalignant skin papilloma in mice. In another study, they also compared the effects of different tea polyphenols on UVB-induced skin carcinogenesis in DMBA-initiated SKH-1 mice using oral administration (Wang et al., 1994). The data showed that oral administration of decaffeinated black tea or decaffeinated green tea had a marked inhibitory effect on UVB-induced skin carcinogenesis in DMBA-initiated SKH-1 mice. Moreover, Meeran et al. (2009) suggested that oral administration of GTPs in drinking water significantly reduced UVB-induced tumor development in wild-type mice. GTPs also resulted in reduction in the levels of markers of inflammation, proliferating cell nuclear antigen, and proinflammatory cytokines in chronically UVB-exposed skin.

3.1.1. Flavonoids

Flavonoids are dietary factors that belong to the general class of compounds known as phytochemicals, or plant chemicals. Flavonoids are gaining international attention for their diverse array of powerful health benefits. Kiefer et al. (2010) found the ideal composition of flavonoids from various citrus extracts for an effective skin lightening cosmetic ingredient. This flavonoid was studied *in vivo* on Caucasian skin for efficacy during 56 days and showed marked skin brightening effects at a concentration of 1%. This liposomal-encapsulated citrus flavonoid blend is effective at 1% in a cosmetic formulation to fade age spots and brighten skin tone. Curcumin is one such phytochemical for which several studies already exist relating its health beneficial effects, mainly as an anti-inflammatory and anti-cancer compound at relatively high dose (Goel et al., 2008). Lima et al. (2011) investigated the effects and molecular mechanisms of action of curcumin on normal human cells undergoing aging. Saija et al. (1998) designed a schedule for a series of *in vivo* experiments, in which the protective effect of topically applied naringenin and hesperetin against UV-B-induced skin damage was assessed monitoring the extent of erythema in human volunteers by means of reflectance spectrophotometry. These findings demonstrate that naringenin and hesperetin may be successfully employed as topical photo-protective agents.

3.1.2. Stilbenes

Stilbenes represent a class of compounds with a common 1, 2-diphenylethylene backbone that have shown extraordinary potential in the biomedical field (Andrei et al., 2014). Silibinin, which is a major component of silymarin, has been shown to inhibit photo-carcinogenesis in mice when applied topically or in the diet (Mallikarjuna et al., 2004). Likewise, the stilbene chemical structure of resveratrol is similar to that synthetic estrogen diethylstilbesterol. The use of phytoestrogens such as resveratrol, are of particular interest since they may provide the skin benefits of estrogen without the associated risks (Farris et al., 2013). Resveratrol is absorbed quickly after oral ingestion with peak plasma levels 30 min after consumption (Goldberg et al., 2003). Kim et al. (2011) showed that oral administration of resveratrol to highly tumor-susceptible p53 (+/-)/SKH-1 mice markedly delayed UV-induced skin tumorigenesis and reduced the malignant conversion of benign papillomas to squamous cell carcinoma. Afaq et al. (2003) have shown that a topical application of resveratrol to SKH-1 hairless mice results in significant inhibitions of UVB-mediated increases in skin edema, inflammation, cyclooxygenase and ornithine decarboxylase induction, and generation of hydrogen peroxide and lipid peroxidation, in the skin. Reagan-Shaw et al (2004) found that repeated UVB exposures resulted in an up-regulation of mitogen activated protein-kinase 1/2 and mitogen-activated protein kinase-1; whereas topical application of resveratrol prior to UVB exposures significantly reversed the UVB-mediated responses in these proteins. Aziz et al. (2005) demonstrated that topical pre-treatment of resveratrol resulted in significant inhibition of UV-B exposure-mediated increases in cellular proliferations, protein levels of epidermal cyclooxygenase-2 (COX-2) and ornithine decarboxylase, established markers of tumor promotion, protein and messenger RNA levels of survivin, and phosphorylation of survivin in the skin of SKH-1 hairless mouse. Bastianetto et al. (2010) found that resveratrol could delay and even prevent the normal course of skin aging by blocking apoptotic events and mitochondrial dysfunctions. Taken together, these findings suggest that resveratrol, by acting on specific polyphenol binding sites in epidermis, may be useful to prevent skin disorders associated with aging.

Moreover, several topical formulations of resveratrol are being developed. Since topical applications are delivered directly to the affected area, this may be an effective approach to combat resveratrols rapid metabolism and allow skin tissue to attain a therapeutic concentration. Studies reported that topical application of resveratrol inhibits UVB-induced skin tumor initiation, promotion and progression (Aziz et al., 2003). In another study, Chen et al. (2006) investigated topical application of resveratrol in a SKH-1 hairless mouse model prior to UV-B irradiation. The results showed that resveratrol lowered levels of ROS in UVA-exposed HaCaT keratinocytes in a dose-dependent manner, and electron microscopy confirmed that ultrastructural changes could be prevented. Hung et al. (2008) have found several different solutions and hydrogel patches as delivery routes for resveratrol. In another study, Kobierski et al. (2009) have tried using several different stabilizers and surfactants to produce a stable nano-suspension of resveratrol, and found that two of the non-ionic stabilizers they worked very well. However, one of the problems is specific to resveratrol's strong photosensitivity. Furthermore, another particular challenge is the stilbene's relatively low water solubility.

3.2. Terpenes

3.2.1. Carotenoids

Carotenoids are organic pigments that are found in the chloroplasts and chromoplasts of plants and some other photosynthetic organisms, including some bacteria and some fungi. *β*-Carotene and astaxanthin are components of carotenoids. Lademann et al . (2011) used resonance Raman spectroscopy to measure the carotenoids non-invasively and online. Carotenoids can serve as marker substances for the complete antioxidative network of human skin. On the other hand, the lycopene concentration in skin also correlates significantly with skin roughness, suggesting that higher levels of antioxidants in the skin effectively decrease skin roughness, which is an early stage of wrinkle formation (Darvin et al., 2008). Moreover, as one of the carotenoids, lutein is the foundation of healthy eyes and skin anti-aging. Highly bioavailable lutein and zeaxanthin in avocado would help to protect the skin from damage from both UV and visible irradiation (Roberts et al., 2009; Dreher and Davenport, 2013). One more study suggested that topical application or oral intake of lutein can provide photo-protective activity (Morganti et al., 2002).

3.2.2. Essential Oils

Essential oils are aromatic oily liquids obtained from plant material (flowers, buds, seeds, leaves, twigs, bark, herbs, wood, fruits and roots) (Burt, 2004). Essential oils are examples of plant products full of vegetal secondary compounds; in fact, secreted by glandular trichomes, they contain the lipophilic fraction of plant phytocomplex and are basically made up of terpenic and phenolic molecules (Angelo et al., 2014). Kim et al. (2009) investigated the anti-elastase activities of the essential oil of air-dried *Illicium anisatum* (IAE). The results indicated that IAE has good anti-elastase effects. Kwon et al. (2013) evaluated essential oil from manuka for its effects against photo-aging in UVB-irradiated hairless mice. The results showed that topical application of manuka essential oil suppressed the UVB-induced increase in skin thickness and wrinkle grading in a dose-dependent manner. Application of 10% manuka essential oil reduced the average length, depth, and % area of wrinkles significantly, and this correlated with inhibition of loss of collagen fiber content and epidermal hyperplasia (Kwon et al., 2013).

3.3. Polysaccharides

Health-promoting *β*-glucans are an auspicious group of polysaccharides, which exhibit a broad spectrum of biological activities including anti-tumor, immune-modulating and anti-inflammatory properties (Du et al., 2015). Furthermore, *β*-glucans have skin health promotion effects. Du et al. (2014) discussed skin health promotion effects of natural beta-glucan derived from cereals and microorganisms. The epidermis contains a large number of macrophages, which can be enhanced and activated in just the same way by a topical *β*-glucan cream. *β*-Glucan is a water-soluble polysaccharide consisting of linear chains of glucose residues with 1, 4 and 1, 3 linkage and has a molecular weight of about 1 million Da. Pillai et al. (2006) conducted a clinical study to evaluate the ability of *β*-glucan to alleviate the extrinsic signs of aging on a panel of 27 subjects with two gel formulations-one with *β*-glucan and the other a placebo. After eight weeks of treatment, a digital image analysis showed that there is a clear improvement in the fine lines and wrinkles of the subjects. They also conducted a moisturisation test on a panel of 30 human subjects with two emulsion formulations-one containing β-glucan and the other with hyaluronic acid. The results showed that β-glucan is an excellent moisturizer and provides even better long-term moisturisation than hyaluronic acid. Moreover, β-glucan modulates wound healing via macrophages, which are stimulated to release growth factors and cytokines, as well as via glucan receptors on fibroblasts, which are activated to migrate and synthesize collagen. The placement of β-glucan/collagen onto an arm of a young child with a scald burn improved healing of a partial-thickness burn wound (Son et al., 2007). Water-soluble carboxymethylated beta-1,3-glucan (CM-glucan) from yeast has gained a lot of interest over the last few years as a new cosmetic ingredient and has been included in many different products on the market. The polysaccharide also non-specifically stimulates the keratinocytes proliferation (Zülli and Suter, 1998) which results in an increase of the renewal rate of the stratum corneum *in vivo* (Zülli et al., 1996). In one study, three oil-in-water emulsions (containing 0.2%, 0.04% and 0% of CM-glucan) were applied twice daily on the forearms of ten volunteers. On the fifth day, the pretreated skin and a non-treated area were exposed to UVA irradiation (10 J/cm^2). An almost complete protection against UVA induced oxidation could be observed in this test with the product containing 0.2% CM-glucan (Zülli et al., 1996). Xie et al. (2008) evaluated the effect of polysaccharides from *Ganoderma lucidum* on the gene expression of keratinocytes to understand the potential mechanisms of *G. lucidum* polysaccharides on delaying aging. In one study, *Hericium erinaceum* polysaccharides significantly enhanced skin antioxidant enzymes, MMP-1, tissue inhibitor of metalloproteinases-1 activities and collagen protein levels in a dose-dependent manner. It can be concluded that *H. erinaceum* polysaccharides possess anti-skin-aging activities (Xu et al., 2010).

3.4. Peptides and Proteins

Collagen, which makes up 75% of the skin, is crucial for the appearance of youthfulness; this naturally-occurring substance makes the skin strong, plump and smooth. Peptides are amino acids that make up the proteins in the skin. They become proteins when they form a long chain of amino acids. Peptides help prevent the visible effects of collagen loss and reduce the appearance of fine lines and wrinkles by working synergistically in serums and creams. They also stimulate collagen and elastin production but are gentler on the dermis. Peptides play a major role in the development of anti aging cosmetics. They occur naturally and are quite often found as messenger proteins and hormones. Also their degradation products, i.e. the amino acids are key players in the field of cosmetic skin care. Cho et al. (2008) investigated the effects of phosphatidylserine on acute UV response and chronologic skin aging by topically applying it to young skin before UV irradiation and to aged human skin, respectively. The results revealed that in the young skin, phosphatidylserine treatment prevented UV-induced reduction in procollagen expression and inhibited UV-induced MMP-1 expression. Phosphatidylserine also blocked UV-induced IL-6 and COX-2 gene expression in cultured fibroblasts dose dependently. Taken together, these results indicated that topical phosphatidylserine has anti-skin-aging properties and point to the potential use of phosphatidylserine as a therapeutic agent in the prevention and treatment of cutaneous aging (Cho et al., 2008). Moreover, a 9-mer peptide, coprisin A3 (CopA3) was synthesized from a natural peptide-coprisin was investigated for its *in vitro* anti-skin photo-aging activity. UV-induced inhibition of type-I procollagen and induction of MMP-1 were partially prevented in human skin fibroblasts by CopA3 peptide in a dose-dependent manner. At a concentration of 25 μM, CopA3 nearly completely inhibited MMP-1 expression. These results suggested that CopA3 is a potential candidate for the prevention and treatment of skin aging (Kim et al., 2014).

It should be mentioned that peptides and proteins are a very complex issue which can only be fragmentarily described. It still has to be clarified whether their use in the anti-aging skin care has consequences on specific interdependent control circuits of the elderly skin and which kind of long term effects will result.

3.5. Saponins

Studies reported that ginseng can activate the skin's metabolism (Tanaka and Okada, 1991), reduce keratinization (Kim et al., 1989), alleviate wrinkling and enhance skin whiteness. Moreover, many studies indicated that the 'antiaging' activity is due to free radical scavenging action of the ginseng saponins (ginsenosides) (Kim et al., 1989). Lee et al. (2007) investigated the possible collagen production-promoting activities of *Panax ginseng* C.A. Meyer root extract (PGRE), mainly saponins. Human Type I procollagen synthesis was also induced by PGRE. When applied topically in a human skin primary irritation test, PGRE did not induce any adverse reactions. These results suggested the possibility that PGRE may be considered as an attractive, wrinkle-reducing candidate for topical application.

3.6. Alkaloids

Kim and Chung (2008) investigated that berberine for capacity to regulate MMP-1 and Type I procollagen expression in human dermal fibroblasts. The results showed that berberine decreased expression of basal and UV-induced MMP-1. Taken together, Type I procollagen expression was dose-dependently increased by berberine. They demonstrate that berberine may be a possible candidate for anti-skin aging agent.

3.7. Phytoestrogen

Phytoestrogens are plant-derived compounds which have biological activities that mimic the effects of estrogen and are used as alternative agents in estrogen therapy (Malaivijitnond, 2012). The chemical structures of phytoestrogens are similar to estrogens in that they have a pair of hydroxyl group and a phenolic ring (Yingngam and Rungseevijitprap, 2012). Lin et al. (2011) investigated the effect of phytoestrogens on collagen synthesis in skin fibroblasts. Among the selected 64 plant extracts and active fractions, soybean isoflavonoids and the ethanol extracts of Radix Puerariae, Spica Humuli Lupuli, Semen Cassiae, Folium Mori and Radix Glycyrrhizae effectively induced the proliferation of MCF-7 cells, but showed no effect on MDA-MB-231 cells. In conclusion, the extracts of Radix Puerariae and soybean isoflavnoids have relatively potent estrogenic activity, suggesting their potential anti-wrinkle and anti-skin aging effect (Li et al., 2011). Moreover, wild yam bio-identical progesterone is progesterone which has been derived from a compound found in Mexican wild yams. It can promote collagen synthesis and improve skin elasticity and moisture retention levels. Barnard (1994) found a cream formulated with wild Mexican yam extract for topical application to be most beneficial. Genistein has many beneficial effects on human health. Wei et al. (2003) discussed the photo-protective effect of genistein in animals and *in vitro* models of human skin. Pretreatment with topical genistein reduced skin roughness and wrinkling and epidermal hyperproliferation in hairless mice that were exposed to daily doses of acute and chronic UVB irradiation. In addition, pretreatment with topical genistein dose-dependently reduced cyclobutane pyrimidine dimers formation and increased proliferating cell nuclear antigen expression in human reconstituted skin samples (Moore et al., 2006).

3.8. Coenzyme Q10

Coenzyme Q10 (CoQ10) is natural compound that was discovered in 1957. Co Q10 may boost skin repair and regeneration and reduce free radical damage. Furthermore, CoQ10 is a small molecule that can relatively easily penetrate into skin cells. In one study, CoQ10 positively influences the age-affected cellular metabolism and enables to combat signs of aging starting at the cellular level. As a consequence topical application of CoQ10 is beneficial for human skin as it rapidly improves mitochondrial function in skin *in vivo* (Prahl et al., 2008).

3.9. Others

Kim et al. (2012) examined the effect of mangiferin isolated from *Anemarrhena asphodeloides* on wrinkle formation, skin thickness, and changes in collagen fibers. In the *in vivo* studies, mangiferin inhibited UVB-induced mean length and mean depth of skin wrinkle based on skin replica, epidermal thickening, and damage to collagen fiber. *L*-Ergothioneine is used as an active ingredient in cosmetics for topical application. This development is strongly supported by the fact that *L*-ergothioneine naturally occurs in skin and is able to counterbalance the effect of key mediators involved in skin aging, and in particular in skin photodamage. Moreover, Emanuele et al. (2014) demonstrated trehalose could reduce UVB-induced corneal damage when topically applied to the eye. Due to the low skin permeability of trehalose, its use as a skin photo-protective agent has been limited. They aimed to assess the protective effects of trehalose-loaded liposomes against UVB-induced photo-damage. The results indicated that trehalose-loaded liposomes showed the highest efficacy in reducing the UVB irradiation. In another study, the effects of piceatannol from passion fruit seed on human keratinocytes were investigated. The pretreatment with piceatannol also suppressed the UVB-induced generation of ROS in the keratinocytes. In addition, the transfer of the medium from the UVB irradiated keratinocytes to non-irradiated fibroblasts enhanced MMP-1 activity, and this MMP-1 induction was reduced when the keratinocytes were pretreated with piceatannol (Maruki-Uchida et al., 2013).

Conclusion and Future Prospective

The science behind skin aging has exploded in the past a few decades. Skin aging has now been defined on both a cellular and molecular level. Developing oral applications of natural products to skin aging could also be an interesting strategy. Clinical trials of cosmeceuticals are important to know the interaction between skin and cosmeceuticals which could even be influenced by environmental factor. And further studies should be performed to assess the potential usefulness in skin photo-protection and the prevention of non-melanoma skin cancer. Although there is potential for natural products as topical photoprotective agents, suitable delivery vehicle, chemical additives, and pH significantly influence the permeation. The efficacy of various topical formulations requires further testing in humans. Taken together, the study of genomics in aging skin provides us with potential targets as points for intervention. At last, further innovation is required to overcome the challenges to effectively deliver natural products into the skin in order to transform the omnipotent extract into a proven therapeutic product.

References

Aburjai, T., Natsheh, F. M. (2003). Plants used in cosmetics. *Phytotherapy Research*, 17, 987-1000.

Afaq, F., Adhami, V. M., Ahmad, N. (2003). Prevention of short-term ultraviolet B radiation-mediated damages by resveratrol in SKH-1 hairless mice. *Toxicology and Applied Pharmacology,* 186, 28-37.

Afaq, F., Katiyar, S. K. (2011). Polyphenols: Skin photo-protection and inhibition of photocarcinogenesis. *Mini-Reviews in Medicinal Chemistry,* 11, 1200-1215.

Andrei, V., Wetie, A. G., Mihai, I., Darie, C. C., Vasilescu, A. (2014). Detection of biomedically relevant stilbenes from wines by mass spectrometry. *Advances in Experimental Medicine and Biology,* 806, 361-382.

Angelo, G., Lorena, C., Marta, G., Antonella, C. (2014). Biochemical composition and antioxidant properties of *Lavandula angustifoli*a Miller essential oil are shielded by propolis against UV radiations. *Photochemistry and Photobiology,* 90, 702-708.

Aziz, M. H., Afaq, F., Ahmad, N. (2005). Prevention of ultraviolet-B radiation damage by resveratrol in mouse skin is mediated via modulation in survivin. *Photochemistry and Photobiology,* 81, 25-31.

Aziz, M. H., Kumar, R., Ahmad, N. (2003). Cancer chemoprevention by resveratrol: *In vitro* and *in vivo* studies and the underlying mechanisms (review). *International Journal of Oncology,* 23, 17-28.

Barnard, N. (1994). Natural progesterone: Is estrogen the wrong hormone? An interview with John R. Lee, M.D. Good Health, Spring Press, pp 11-13.

Bastianetto, S., Dumont, Y., Duranton, A., Vercauteren, F., Breton, L., Quirion, R. (2010). Protective action of resveratrol in human skin: Possible involvement of specific receptor binding sites. *PLoS One,* 5, e12935.

Baxter, R. A. (2008). Anti-aging properties of resveratrol: Review and report of a potent new antioxidant skin care formulation. *Journal of Cosmetic Dermatology,* 7, 2-7.

Baumann, L. (2002). Cosmetic dermatology. New York: McGraw-Hill Press, pp 226.

Baumann, L. (2007). Skin ageing and its treatment. *Journal of Pathology,* 211, 241-251.

Burt, S. (2004). Essential oils: Their antibacterial properties and potential applications in foods-a review. *International Journal of Food Microbiology,* 94, 223-253.

Chen, M. L., Li, J., Xiao, W. R., Sun, L., Tang, H., Wang, L., Wu, L. Y., Chen, X., Xie, H. F. (2006). Protective effect of resveratrol against oxidative damage of UVA irradiated HaCaT cells. *Journal of Central South University (Medical Science),* 31, 635-639.

Cho, S., Kim. H. H., Lee, M. J., Lee, S., Park, C. S., Nam, S. J., Han, J. J., Kim, J. W., Chung, J. H. (2008). Phosphatidylserine prevents UV-induced decrease of Type I procollagen and increase of MMP-1 in dermal fibroblasts and human skin *in vivo*. *Journal of Lipid Research,* 49, 1235-1245.

Chondrogianni, N., Kapeta, S., Chinou, I., Vassilatou, K., Papassideri, I., Gonos, E. S. (2010). Anti-ageing and rejuvenating effects of quercetin. *Experimental Gerontology,* 45, 763-771.

Darvin, M., Patzelt, A., Gehse, S., Schanzer, S., Benderoth, C., Sterry, W., Lademann, J. (2008). Cutaneous concentration of lycopene correlates significantly with the roughness of the skin. *European Journal of Pharmaceutics and Biopharmaceutics,* 69, 943-947.

Dreher, M. L., Davenport, A. J. (2013). Hass avocado composition and potential health effects. *Critical Reviews in Food Science and Nutrition*, 53, 738-750.

Du, B., Lin, C. Y., Bian, Z. X., Xu, B. J. (2015). An insight into anti-inflammatory effects of fungal beta-glucans. *Trends in Food Science and Technology*, 41, 49-59.

Du, B., Bian, Z. X., Xu, B. J. (2014). Skin health promotion effects of natural beta-glucan derived from cereals and microorganisms: A review. *Phytotherapy Research*, 28, 159-166.

Emanuele, E., Bertona, M., Sanchis-Gomar, F., Pareja-Galeano, H., Lucia, A. (2014). Protective effect of trehalose-loaded liposomes against UVB-induced photodamage in human keratinocytes. *Biomedical Reports,* 2, 755-759.

Farris, P., Krutmann, J., Li, Y. H., McDaniel, D., Krol, Y. (2013). Resveratrol: A unique antioxidant offering a multi-mechanistic approach for treating aging skin. *Journal of Drugs in Dermatology,* 12, 1389-1394.

Goel, A., Kunnumakkara, A. B., Aggarwal, B. B. (2008). Curcumin as "Curecumin": From kitchen to clinic. *Biochemical Pharmacology,* 75, 787-809.

Goldberg, D. M., Yan, J., Soleas, G. J. (2003). Absorption of three wine-related polyphenols in three different matrices by healthy subjects. *Clinical Biochemistry,* 36, 79-87.

Grace, R. (2002). Cosmeceuticals: Functional food for the skin. Natural Foods Merchandiser XXIII, 92-99.

Hung, C. F., Lin, Y. K., Huang, Z. R., Fang, J. Y. (2008). Delivery of resveratrol, a red wine polyphenol, from solutions and hydrogels via the skin. *Biological and Pharmaceutical Bulletin,* 31, 955-962.

Jeon, H. Y., Kim, J. K., Kim, W. G., Lee, S. J. (2009). Effects of oral epigallocatechin gallate supplementation on the minimal erythema dose and UV-induced skin damage. *Skin Pharmacology and Physiology,* 22, 137-141.

Katiyar, S. K., Matsui, M. S., Elmets, C. A., Mukhtar, H. (1999). Polyphenolic antioxidant (-)-epigallocatechin-3-gallate from green tea reduces UVB-induced inflammatory responses and infiltration of leukocytes in human skin. *Photochemistry and Photobiology,* 69, 148-153.

Khavkin,J., Ellis, D. A. F. (2011). Aging skin: Histology, physiology, and pathology. *Facial Plastic Surgery Clinics of North America,* 19, 229-234.

Kiefer, S., Weibel, M., Smits, J., Juch, M., Tiedtke, J., Herbst, N. (2010). Citrus flavonoids with skin lightening effects-safety and efficacy studies. *SOFW Journal,* 136, 46-54.

Kim, D. H., Kim, H. H., Kim, H. J., Jung, H. G., Yu, J. M., Lee, E. S., Cho, Y. H., Kim, D. I., An, B. J. (2014). CopA3 peptide prevents ultraviolet-induced inhibition of type-I procollagen and induction of matrix metalloproteinase-1 in human skin fibroblasts. *Molecules,* 19, 6407-6414.

Kim, H. Y., Jin, S.H., Kim, S. I. (1989). Effect of 1, 3-*cis*-retinoic acid and ginseng saponin on hyperkeratinization of guinea pig skin. *Koryo Insam Hakhoe chi*, 13, 248-253.

Kim, H. S., Song, J. H., Youn, U. J., Hyun, J. W., Jeong, W. S., Lee, M. Y., Choi, H. J., Lee, H. K., Chae, S. (2012). Inhibition of UVB-induced wrinkle formation and MMP-9 expression by mangiferin isolated from *Anemarrhena asphodeloides*. *European Journal of Pharmacology,* 689, 38-44.

Kim, J. Y., Kim, S. S., Oh, T. H., Baik, J. S., Song, G., Lee, N. H., Hyun, C. G. (2009). Chemical composition, antioxidant, anti-elastase, and anti-inflammatory activities of *Illicium anisatum* essential oil. *Acta Pharmaceutica*, 59, 289-300.

Kim, K. H., Back, J. H., Zhu, Y., Arbesman, J., Athar, M., Kopelovich, L., Kim, A. L., Bickers, D. R. (2011). Resveratrol targets transforming growth factor-β2 signaling to block UV-induced tumor progression. *Journal of Investigative Dermatology,* 131, 195-202.

Kim, S., Chung, J. H. (2008). Berberine prevents UV-induced MMP-1 and reduction of Type I procollagen expression in human dermal fibroblasts. *Phytomedicine*, 15, 749-753.

Kobierski, S., Ofori-Kwakye, K., Muller, R. H., Keck, C. M. (2009). Resveratrol nanosuspensions for dermal application--production, characterization, and physical stability. *Pharmazie,* 64, 741-747.

Kosmadaki, M. G., Gilchrest, B. A. (2004). The role of telomeres in skin aging/photoaging. *Micron,* 35, 155-159.

Krutmann, J., Schroeder, P. (2009). Role of mitochondria in photoaging of human skin: The defective powerhouse model. *Journal of Investigative Dermatology Symposium Proceedings*, 14, 44-49.

Kwon, O. S., Jung, S. H., Yang, B. S. (2013). Topical administration of manuka oil prevents UV-B irradiation-induced cutaneous photoaging in mice. *Evidence-Based Complementary and Alternative Medicine,* 2013, 1-11.

Lademann, J., Meinke, M. C., Sterry, W., Darvin, M. E. (2011). Carotenoids in human skin. *Experimental Dermatology,* 20, 377-382.

Lall, N., Kishore, N. (2014). Are plants used for skin care in South Africa fully explored? *Journal of Ethnopharmacology,* 153, 61-84.

Langton, A. K., Sherratt, M. J., Griffiths, C. E. M., Watson, R. E. B. (2010). A new wrinkle on old skin: The role of elastic fibres in skin ageing. *International Journal of Cosmetic Science,* 32, 330-339.

Lee, J., Jung, E., Lee, J., Huh, S., Kim, J., Park, M., So, J., Ham, Y., Jung, K., Hyun, C. G., Kim, Y. S., Park, D. (2007). *Panax ginseng* induces human Type I collagen synthesis through activation of Smad signaling. *Journal of Ethnopharmacology,* 109, 29-34.

Li, L., Qu, X. T., Lu, Yang. (2011). Screening for phytoestrogens and their anti-skin aging effect *in vitro. Journal of Shanghai Jiaotong University (Medical Science),* 31, 1361-1365.

Lima, C. F., Pereira-Wilson, C., Rattan, S. I. (2011). Curcumin induces heme oxygenase-1 in normal human skin fibroblasts through redox signaling: Relevance for anti-aging intervention. *Molecular Nutrition and Food Research,* 55, 430-442.

Malaivijitnond, S. (2012). Medical applications of phytoestrogens from the Thai herb *Pueraria mirifica. Frontiers of Medicine*, 6, 8-21.

Mallikarjuna, G., Dhanalakshmi, S., Singh, R. P., Agarwal, C., Agarwal, R. (2004). Silibinin protects against photocarcinogenesis via modulation of cell cycle regulators, mitogen-activated protein kinases, and Akt signaling. *Cancer Research,* 64, 6349-6356.

Maruki-Uchida, H., Kurita, I., Sugiyama, K., Sai, M., Maeda, K., Ito, T. (2013). The protective effects of piceatannol from passion fruit (*Passiflora edulis*) seeds in UVB-irradiated keratinocytes. *Biological and Pharmaceutical Bulletin,* 36, 845-849.

Masaki, H. (2010). Role of antioxidants in the skin: Anti-aging effects. *Journal of Dermatological Science,* 58, 85-90.

Meeran, S. M., Akhtar, S., Katiyar, S. K. (2009). Inhibition of UVB-induced skin tumor development by drinking green tea polyphenols is mediated through DNA repair and subsequent inhibition of inflammation. *Journal of Investigative Dermatology,* 129, 1258-1270.

Mittal, A., Piyathilake, C., Hara, Y., Katiyar, S. K. (2003). Exceptionally high protection of photocarcinogenesis by topical application of (--)-epigallocatechin-3-gallate in hydrophilic cream in SKH-1 hairless mouse model: Relationship to inhibition of UVB-induced global DNA hypomethylation. *Neoplasia,* 5, 555-565.

Moore, J. O., Wang, Y., Stebbins, W. G., Gao, D., Zhou, X., Phelps, R., Lebwohl, M., Wei, H. (2006). Photoprotective effect of isoflavone genistein on ultraviolet B-induced pyrimidine dimer formation and PCNA expression in human reconstituted skin and its implications in dermatology and prevention of cutaneous carcinogenesis. *Carcinogenesis,* 27, 1627-1635.

Morganti, P., Bruno, C., Guarneri, F., Cardillo, A., Del Ciotto, P. and Valenzano, F. (2002). Role of topical and nutritional supplement to modify the oxidative stress. *International Journal of Cosmetic Science,* 24, 331-339.

Mukherjee, P. K., Maity, N., Nema, N. K., Sarkar, B. K. (2011). Bioactive compounds from natural resources against skin aging. *Phytomedicine,* 19, 64-73.

Mukul, S., Surabhi, K., Atul, N. (2011). Cosmeceuticals for the skin: An overview. *Asian Journal of Pharmaceutical and Clinical Research,* 4, 1-6.

Ndiaye, M., Philippe, C., Mukhtar, H., Ahmad, N. (2011). The grape antioxidant resveratrol for skin disorders: Promise, prospects, and challenges. *Archives of Biochemistry and Biophysics,* 508, 164-170.

Nichols, J. A., Katiyar, S. K. (2010). Skin photoprotection by natural polyphenols: Anti-inflammatory, anti-oxidant and DNA repair mechanisms. *Archives of Dermatological Research,* 302, 71-83.

Perricone, N. (2001). The wrinkle cure. New York: Warner Books; 207 p.

Pillai, R., Röding, J., Redmond, M. (2006). Beta-glucan - A multi-functional skin care active. Cosmetic Science and Technology, 140.

Prahl, S., Kueper, T., Biernoth, T., Wöhrmann, Y., Münster, A., Fürstenau, M., Schmidt, M., Schulze, C., Wittern, K. P., Wenck, H., Muhr, G. M., Blatt, T. (2008). Aging skin is functionally anaerobic: Importance of coenzyme Q10 for anti aging skin care. *Biofactors,* 32, 245-255.

Puizina-Ivić, N. (2008). Skin aging. *Acta Dermatovenerol Alp Pannonica Adriat,* 17, 47-54.

Reagan-Shaw, S., Afaq, F., Aziz, M. H., Ahmad, N. (2004). Modulations of critical cell cycle regulatory events during chemoprevention of ultraviolet B-mediated responses by resveratrol in SKH-1 hairless mouse skin. *Oncogene,* 23, 5151-5160.

Roberts, R. L., Green, J., Lewis, B. (2009). Lutein and zeaxanthin in eye and skin health. *Clinics in Dermatology,* 27, 195-201.

Saija, A., Tomaino, A., Trombetta, D., Giacchi, M., De Pasquale, A., Bonina, F. (1998). Influence of different penetration enhancers on *in vitro* skin permeation and *in vivo* photoprotective effect of flavonoids. *International Journal of Pharmaceutics,* 175, 85-94.

Sander, C. S., Chang, H., Salzmann, S., Müller, C. S., Ekanayake-Mudiyanselage, S., Elsner, P., Thiele, J. J. (2002). Photoaging is associated with protein oxidation in human skin *in vivo*. *Journal of Investigative Dermatology,* 118, 618-625.

Schagen, S. K., Zampeli, V. A., Makrantonaki, E., Zouboulis, C. C. (2012). Discovering the link between nutrition and skin aging. *Dermato-Endocrinology,* 4, 298-307.

Son, H. J., Han, D. W., Baek, H. S., Lim, H. R., Lee, M. H., Woo, Y. I., Park, J. C. (2007). Stimulated TNF-α release in macrophage and enhanced migration of dermal fibroblast by β-glucan. *Current Applied Physics,* 7S1, e33-e36.

Tanaka, H., Okada, T. (1991). Effect of *Panax ginseng* on the production of glycosaminoglycans in cultured human skin fibroblast. *Frag Journal,* 19, 90-91.

Tanaka, Y. T., Tanaka, K., Kojima, H., Hamada, T., Masutani, T., Tsuboi, M., Akao, Y. (2013). Cynaropicrin from *Cynara scolymus* L. suppresses photoaging of skin by inhibiting the transcription activity of nuclear factor-kappa B. *Bioorganic and Medicinal Chemistry Letters,* 23, 518-523.

Varani, J. (2010). Fibroblast aging: Intrinsic and extrinsic factors. *Drug Discovery Today: Therapeutic Strategies,* 7, 65-70.

Wang, Z. Y., Huang, M. T., Ho, C. T., Chang, R., Ma, W., Ferraro, T., Reuhl, K. R., Yang, C. S., Conney, A. H. (1992). Inhibitory effect of green tea on the growth of established skin papillomas in mice. *Cancer Research,* 52, 6657-6665.

Wang, Z. Y., Huang, M. T., Lou, Y. R., Xie, J. G., Reuhl, K. R., Newmark, H. L., Ho, C. T., Yang, C. S., Conney, A. H. (1994). Inhibitory effects of black tea, green tea, decaffeinated black tea, and decaffeinated green tea on ultraviolet B light-induced skin carcinogenesis in 7,12-dimethylbenz[a]anthracene-initiated SKH-1 mice. *Cancer Research,* 54, 3428-3435.

Wei, H., Saladi, R., Lu, Y., Wang, Y., Palep, S. R., Moore, J., Phelps, R., Shyong, E., Lebwohl, M. G. (2003). Isoflavone genistein: Photoprotection and clinical implications in dermatology. *Journal of Nutrition,* 133, 3811S-3819S.

Xie, S. Q., Liao, W. Q., Yao, Z. R., Wang, Z. D. (2008). Related gene expressions in anti-keratinocyte aging induced by *Ganoderma lucidum* polysaccharides. *Journal of Medical Colleges of PLA*, 23, 167-175.

Xu, H., Wu. P. R., Shen, Z. Y., Chen, X. D. (2010). Chemical analysis of *Hericium erinaceum* polysaccharides and effect of the polysaccharides on derma antioxidant enzymes, MMP-1 and TIMP-1 activities. *International Journal of Biological Macromolecules,* 47, 33-36.

Yingngam, B., Rungseevijitprapa, W. (2012). Molecular and clinical role of phytoestrogens as anti-skin-ageing agents: A critical overview. *Phytopharmacology,* 3, 227-244

Zülli, F., Suter, F. (1998). Improving skin function with CM-glucan, a biological response modifier from yeast. *International Journal of Cosmetic Science,* 20, 79-86.

Zülli, F., Suter, F., Biltz, H., Nissen, H.P., Birman, M. (1996). Carboxymethylated beta-(1,3)-glucan. *Cosmetics and Toiletries,* 111, 91-98.

In: Skin Aging and Photoaging
Editor: Emanuel Graham

ISBN: 978-1-63482-907-6

Chapter 2

Equol: A Botanical Active Ingredient for Human Skin Anti-aging

Edwin D. Lephart*
Department of Physiology and Developmental Biology,
The Neuroscience Center, College of Life Sciences,
Brigham Young University, Provo, Utah, US

Abstract

A brief review of skin characteristics (epi-, dermis, and hypo-dermal components), skin aging mechanisms (extrinsic or photo-aging vs. intrinsic or chronological aging), dermal applications [moisturizers, hormone/estrogen replacement therapies- (HRT & ERT), etc.], steroid actions in human skin [estrogens and androgens such as dihydrotestosterone (5α-DHT)], steroid enzymes in human skin (5α-reductase) and steroid receptors in human skin [estrogen receptors (ERs), androgen receptors (ARs) and estrogen-related receptors (ERRs) are important to understand in reference to skin aging. Skin aging is an important clinical topic with facial wrinkling having top priority. The basic biology of human skin aging is dependent upon a host of factors (photoexposure, muscle contraction, chronological aging and environmental agents). Collagen and elastin play essential roles in

* Corresponding author: Telephone 801 422 2006, Fax 801 422 0700.

optimal skin health. Chronological changes lead to temporary wrinkles that directly evolve into persistent wrinkles (especially, "crow's feet" around the eyes). The rate of wrinkle formation accelerates in middle-aged women, but since this process appears to begin in the twenties, practicing regular skin care should begin early. The goal is to delay aging onset and slow down or reverse the rate of wrinkling with time. This can be accomplish with some cosmeticeuticals or phytochemical (botanticals) that increase collagen and elastin while at the same time inhibit the enzymes (matrix metalloproteinases that breakdown, collagen & elastin). The term cosmeceutical has beneficial biological effects that overlap with phytochemical (or botanical) treatments that are being introduced into cosmetic products. One emerging botanical is a polyphenolic (isoflavonoid) molecule (i.e., equol) that has been shown to improve human skin health that can be incorporated into clinical practice. Specifically, equol's characteristics (chemical structure, steroid binding characteristics and isomeric expression) are presented followed by human skin *in vitro* (basic science) and *in vivo* (clinical) studies. Moreover, since equol is expressed as isomers, the youthful expression of dermal genes/proteins via equol demonstrate how: a) R-equol and/or Racemic equol are better molecules for dermal gene and protein expression in anti-aging effects compared to S-equol, and thus would be more efficacious ingredients in topical applications and b) the reservoir forming properties of equol in the epidermis are due to its lipophilic characteristics and/or its affinity for estrogen receptor subtypes allowing for novel delivery of its positive actions to improve skin health and regeneration. Finally, various mechanisms/pathways [increases of collagen, elastin, tissue inhibitor of matrix metalloproteinase (TIMP) and decreases in matrix metalloproteinases (MMPs), inflammatory molecules and 5α-reductase] via reactive oxygen species (ROS), oxidative stress, binding to 5α-DHT, ERs and ERRs and activation of nuclear-factor-erythroid 2-related factor 2 (Nrf2) explain how equol functions as a botanical active ingredient in human skin as an effective anti-aging dermal treatment.

Human Skin Biology

Human skin is the largest and most complex organ (representing one sixth of the total body weight) [1] functioning as a physical barrier to protect the body from water loss as well as environmental insults such as pathogens, chemicals, physical agents and solar ultraviolet radiation (UVR) throughout life [1, 2]. Moreover, the skin provides essential physiological functions including immune defense, thermoregulation, sensory input from mechanoreceptors and endocrine and metabolic mechanisms to sustain optimal health [2].

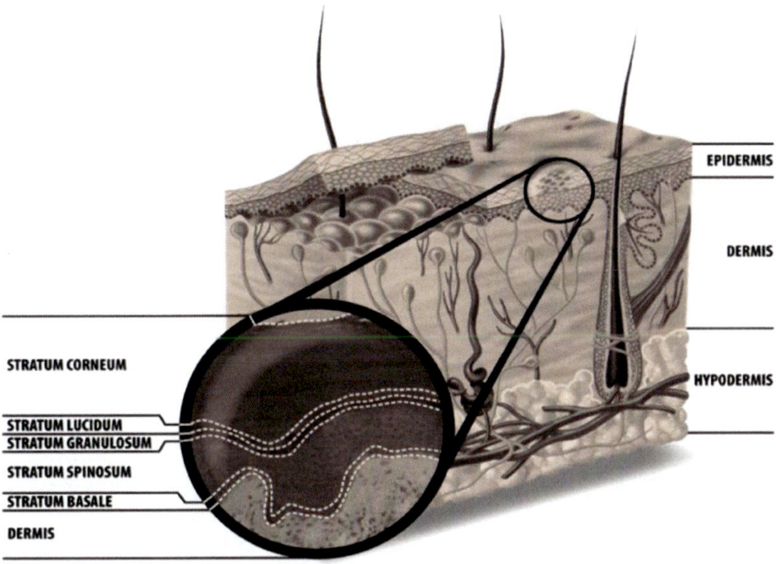

Figure 1. A cartoon graphic displaying the three skin layers in humans. The circle at the epidermal/dermal junction is enlarged showing epidermal cell layers and the upper portion of the dermis. Note: the stratum lucidum is present only in glabrous skin (palmar- palms of the hands and plantar- soles of the feet).

The skin is divided into three distinct layers: 1) the epidermis; 2) the dermis; and 3) the hypodermis or subcutaneous tissue [2]. See Figure 1 for a basic graphic representation of the human skin layers.

Epidermis

The epidermis is the major protective outer layer with keratinocytes as the major cell type [2]. The epidermis (100-150 microns thick) is stratified further into 4 distinct layers with the stratum corneum forming the outermost seal or layer composed of approximately 15-20 cell layers (or 10-30 microns in thickness) and lipids [3]. The brick and mortar structure is a classic model for the organization of the stratum corneum where the "bricks" are the multiple layers of protein-enriched dead corneocytes (approximately 60%) tightly packed with a surrounding covering that serves as the "mortar" composed of hydrophobic lipids (20%) that gives the skin physical protection against water loss, pathogens, and other chemicals or molecules [4]. It should be noted that the water content of the stratum corneum (about 20%) is much lower compared to the other epidermal layers (at about 70%) with a sharp drop at the stratum corneum and stratum granulosum junction [5].

Dermis

The dermis is a dense and irregular layer of connective tissue, 2 to 3 mm thick, that comprises most of the skin thickness [6]. The epidermal-dermal junction is denoted by the basement membrane of the basal cells or stratum germinativum in the epidermis [7]. The epidermis is devoid of a blood supply while the vasculature of the dermis contains much of the skin's blood supply [5]. It also contains free nerve endings, mechanosensory receptors, sweat and oil (sebaceous) glands, and its primary water-holding components i.e., hyaluronic acid (responsible for normal turgor) and supportive glycosaminoglycans that support optimal skin health [5, 7]. The dermis is also responsible for controlling the pH of the skin. It is composed mainly of extracellular matrix proteins (such as collagen, elastin, etc.) that are secreted by fibroblasts and provide for the structural or scaffolding components of the skin for dermal strength and flexibility. The collagen fibers contribute most of the mass of the skin and the bulk of its tensile strength [2]. The elastic fiber network is responsible for recoil and elasticity of the skin [8]. The dermal layer also contain other molecules such as tissue inhibitor of matrix metalloproteinases (TIMP), metalloproteinases, elastase and many other molecules that maintain skin health [5]. Finally, the dermis serves as a connective layer to the epidermis and binds all above layers to the hypodermis [1, 5].

Hypodermis

The hypodermis is a layer of loose connective tissue below the dermis. [Since most of the treatment, biological and functional actions take place in the epidermis and dermis for cosmetic applications only a brief description of the hypodermis is presented here.] The hypodermis contains larger blood vessels and provides for thermoregulation, subcutaneous fat (for energy storage, insulation and cushioning), areolar connective tissue and stabilizes the skin by connecting the dermis to internal organs [5, 7, 9].

Pathology of Skin Aging

Aging is accompanied by the progressive loss of anatomical structure and physiological function in multiple organs. According to recent statistics, approximately 25% of Americans are expected to be 65 years old or older by the year 2030 [10]. Furthermore, in Western countries it is estimated that women will spend more than one-third of their lifetimes in post menopause [6] and more than 40 million postmenopausal women live in the USA today, composing 17% of the total population [11]. Thus, it is important to understand the skin aging process and accompanying anatomical/physiological changes for medical reasons and for personal care perception of optimal dermal health. For the individual loss of youthful appearance have important social and self-perception implications.

As human beings age, the skin thins, dries, wrinkles, and becomes unevenly pigmented [12] and the skin displays delayed wound healing [8]. There is loss of subcutaneous fat, as well as underlying bone and cartilage that leads to sagging skin [13]. In fact, skin complaints by older adults, particularly women, are largely esthetic and plastic surgery has become one of the fasting growing medical specialties [12]. However, aging of the skin can also produce morbidity since most people over 65 have at least one skin disorder [14]. This focus on skin aging highlights the efforts for cutaneous medical care and cosmetic improvements to increase the quality of life for a growing population of aging adults. Remarkably: because, there is not a clear line of distinction between medical concerns/procedures in dermatology and cosmetic applications both strive to assist patients to look good so they in turn can feel better about themselves. For example, whether a person goes through dermal trauma from war or accidental means compared to individuals experiencing chronological skin aging the impact on patients in regard to positive self-perception is paramount especially if the events/changes occur in highly visible body areas such as the face, neck, hands and arm-regions.

Skin aging can be classified by intrinsic and extrinsic process [15]. The intrinsic or chronological aging includes several factors such as genetics, metabolism and the passage of time where the "repair process" may become defective [16]. The repair process is an important component with aging since DNA and the gene products, proteins play such an essential role in optimal dermal health. On the other hand, extrinsic aging is caused by environmental exposure, primarily UVR or ultra violet (UV) light and this is more commonly termed photoaging. The UV light (UVC, UVB and UVA) characteristics pertaining to human skin photoaging and damage are displayed in Figure 2. In sun-exposed skin areas, photoaging involves changes in cellular activities that lead to gross disorganization of the dermal matrix [17]. For example, within the dermis fibroblasts contribute to the production of many extracellular matrix proteins such as collagen, elastin, elastase, matrix metaolloproteinases (MMPs), tissue inhibitors of metalloproteinases (TIMPs) and other molecules such as anti-oxidants and anti-aging factors that are important for maintaining healthy skin [18-20].

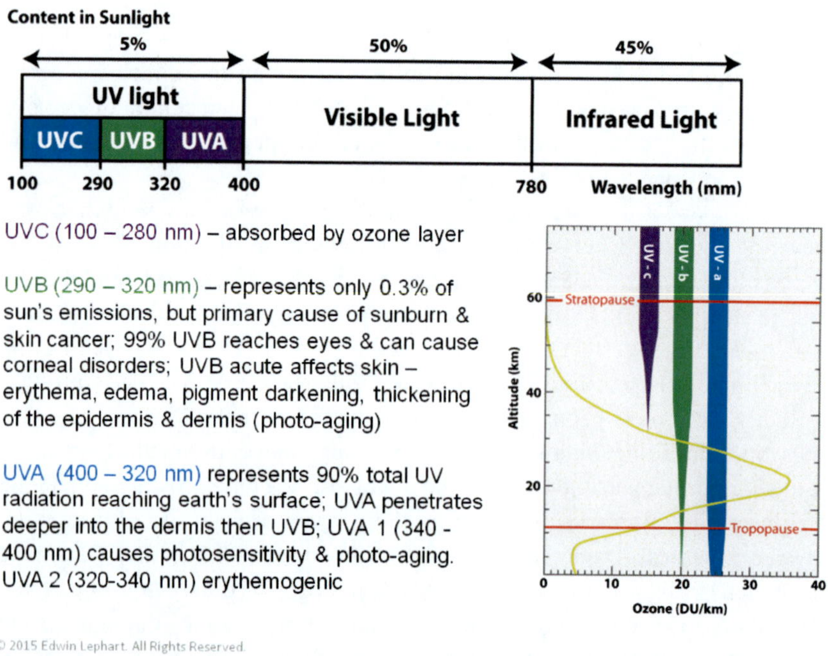

Figure 2. The solar radiation spectrum and the influences of ultra violet (UV) light on skin aging. Brief descriptions of UVC, UVB and UVA characteristics are shown especially in reference to specific amounts and patterns of UV penetration into the skin and the potential damage each can cause with exposure.

Notably, skin collagen peaks around 30 years of age [18, 19], which corresponds with the peak of estrogen production around 25-30 years of age [21, 22] (see Figure 3). The first signs of skin aging occur around age 30 and especially after menopause where there is skin dryness, decreased skin firmness and loss of elasticity [18, 19]. In fact, elasticity has been shown (via mechanical depression) to be highest in young (10 year old) subjects with a continual gradual decline with chronological aging [23] (see Figure 3). However, topical moisturizers with validated active ingredients and/or estrogen or oral hormone replacement therapy (ERT/HRT) have been shown to improve skin aging parameters and reverse the negative effects of skin aging compared to untreated skin [18, 20].

For extrinsic aging, exposure to the sun or photoaging results in many events that lead to the production of endogenous reactive oxygen species (ROS) that in turn increase the production of matrix metalloproteinases (MMPs) that breakdown the important collagen dermal fibers and also can breakdown elastin [17]. These insults can lead to dermal fibroblast collapse that in turn will speed up the process of intrinsic aging with the generation of wrinkles [17] (see Figure 4). For all individuals the aging mechanisms are continually in play and the dermatological focus must be on decreasing or slowing down the aging of the skin by increasing collagen and elastin components while at the same time decreasing the production of MMPs (that breakdown collagen and elastin) [24].

Clinical Signs of Facial Wrinkling

In the examination of aging skin, facial wrinkling is the highest profile topic [25]. The principle sites of facial wrinkles are "crow's feet" around the eye, transverse forehead lines, glabellar frown lines and the nasolabial folds with aging. These kinds of wrinkles can be either temporary or persistent. Temporary lines form in the skin during the process of muscle contraction and disappear when the facial muscles relax. Conversely, persistent wrinkles are visible at rest without muscle contraction. These wrinkles are a result of muscle contractions associated most often with smiling where emotional expressions are produced by 43 unique facial muscles that can produce over 10,000 facial movements [25]. The primary function of facial muscles is to move skin. Notably, the orbicularis oculi around the orbit of the eye, when contracted with smiling, produces characteristic "crow's feet" wrinkles, which suggests that smiling produces temporary lines that become persistent with aging (see below).

Of course, UV-induced skin damage is an accelerator of facial wrinkling. Also, the role of elastin and collagen in cutaneous aging has been validated [26]. However, a recent study has clearly demonstrated that the age-related loss in skin elasticity actually precedes the formation of visible wrinkles by about 20 years [27]. The loss of facial skin mechanical properties starts very early in life, earlier than one might expect, perhaps even as early as 10-15 years of age [23]. Thus, the importance of practicing good skin care habits (i.e., the use of sunscreens and moisturizers) from early childhood is recommended in order to best retain the skin's youthful elastic qualities, and thereby, delay the onset and decrease the severity of wrinkling with aging.

Estrogen, Collagen, Elasticity and Aging

- Estrogen levels peak around the late 20s
- Skin collagen/elastin peaks at approximately age 30 in women, then declines, corresponding to lack of estrogen
- Elasticity decreases with increasing age

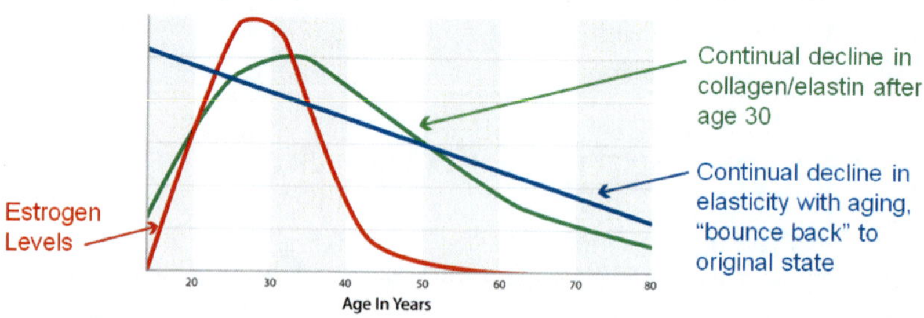

 1

Figure 3. Production of estrogen, collagen/elastin and elasticity profiles/patterns in women with age. Estrogen levels peak in the late twenties, while collagen and elastin peak around age 30. Elasticity is greatest in very young individuals (10 year olds), which continually decline with age.

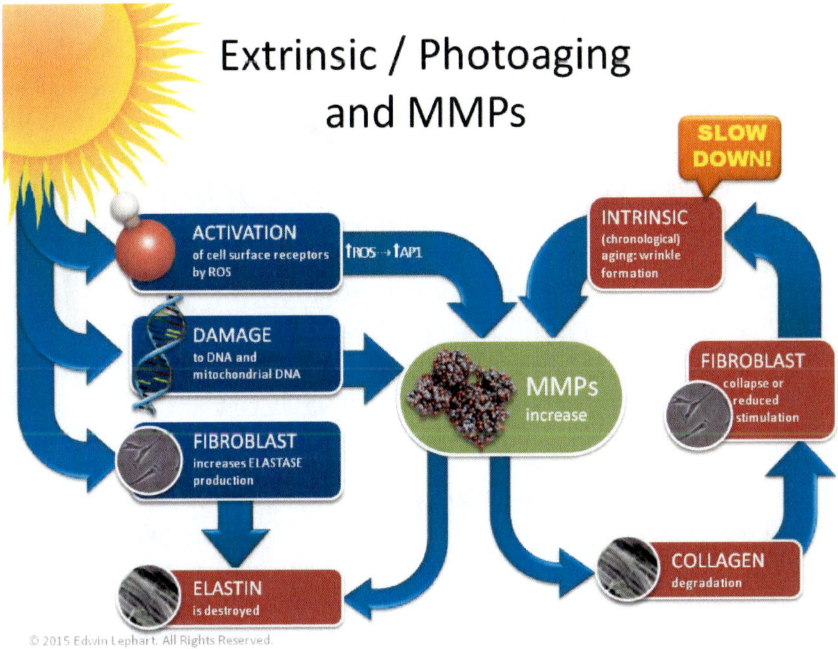

Figure 4. Extrinsic/Photoaging caused by solar radiation (UV light) and the stimulation of matrix metaloproteinases (MMPs) by various pathways, which break down collagen and elastin. Reactive oxygen species (ROS), activator protein 1 (AP1). The goal is to slow down wrinkle formation from photoaging.

In the 1990s a proposal was put forth to consider how the skin's architecture deteriorates with aging with the concomitant loss of elasticity, making the skin less able to rebound from repeated mechanical stress or contraction. To test this hypothesis a study was conducted where subjects were imaged for facial wrinkling in a relaxed or neutral state versus a smiling expression that accentuated crow's feet around the eyes [28]. Using facial imaging analysis examining over 4,000 women on both the left and right sides of the face yielded wrinkle severity for each subject where persistent wrinkling was observed from non-smiling expressions and temporary wrinkling was quantified from the smiling images. This technique demonstrated that the smiling expression yielded more wrinkle lines compared to the non-smiling expression.

In another study conducted in China, facial wrinkling was assessed in 450 normal healthy women that ranged in age from 10 to 70 years old (or 75 subjects per decade) [29]. In the youth age group (ages 10-19) both temporary and persistent facial wrinkles are largely absent. However, in early adult life (typically in their twenties), the first signs of wrinkling show as temporary lines during facial expression whereas, persistent wrinkles are still largely absent. Thus, depending on a person's exposure to the sun and other factors determines when, persistent facial wrinkles will start to appear [29].

To determine how important extrinsic aging factors are in facial wrinkle formation, image analysis was performed examining monozygotic ("identical") twins. Since each twin pair has an identical chromosomal DNA sequence and since most twins are raised in the same households and exposed to similar environments, similar severities of wrinkling between the twins were expected, and this is exactly what was found [25]!

Next, to track the progression of individual lines and wrinkles on a given subject an 8 year study was performed [30]. Each subject's pattern of wrinkling around the eyes and on the cheek, with and without smiling, at baseline was compared to the pattern observed after 8 years. It was found that a subject's unique pattern of persistent facial wrinkling with a neutral expression at 8 years was predicted by the pattern of temporary wrinkling seen with a smiling expression at baseline. Thus, the repeated mechanical flexure along the same skin lines causes temporary lines to eventually become persistent wrinkles. With respect to the influence of age on the rate of wrinkling, the study found that subjects, who were in their forties at baseline, displayed a significantly faster rate of wrinkling over the 8-year period compared to women in other age groups at baseline [30], confirming the results of other studies showing increased rate of skin wrinkling during middle age for women [31, 32]. Finally, the relationship of menopausal status and rate of wrinkling was examined. Women, who had entered menopause between baseline and 8 years, showed the highest rate of wrinkling (> 95% increase), and the observation that hormone replacement therapy did not improve skin wrinkling in women, who were 5 years postmenopausal was consistent with previous reports [33].

Aging simulation studies have identified how people, who are naturally curious, will look, in 5, 10 years for more years. It is known that each person has their own aging skin "destiny," and the challenge is to simulation facial aging as accurately as possible. Current image-based computer simulation models can now accurately depict how facial aging will take place based upon the fact that temporary wrinkles observed with smiling are predictive of future persistent wrinkles [25]. By capturing images of a person with a neutral (non-smiling) expression followed by imaging the same person with a smiling expression, then morphing the temporary wrinkles from the smiling expression image onto the neutral image, the resulting image will simulate future persistent wrinkling in a unique pattern and severity to that particular individual.

Importance of Skin Steroid Receptors, Steroid Enzymes and Steroid Hormones in Aging

The most important steroid receptors in skin are estrogen and androgen receptors. Estrogen receptors (ER) are expressed as subtypes, estrogen receptor alpha (ER α) and estrogen receptor beta (ER β; see Figure 5). The predominant subtype of ER in skin and scalp hair is ER β, in keratinocytes, fibroblasts and the hair bulb [24]. Androgen receptors (AR) are expressed at lower levels compared to ER β in fibroblasts in the dermis [24]. The ER β and androgen receptors play important roles in the skin and hair health. In general, activation of ER β enhances, whereas, activation of androgen receptors decreases skin and hair health.

Also, the 5α-reductase enzyme is present in fibroblasts. This enzyme converts testosterone to the more potent androgen, 5α-dihydrotestosterone (5α-DHT) that decreases skin fibroblast cell viability and wound healing [24] (see Figure 5). Finally, estrogen related receptor (ERR) gamma (γ) has been identified in human skin that has positive influences on dermal health [34] (see below).

Slowing down the Fast Moving Train of Skin Aging and Facial Wrinkle Development

Aging can be described as a fast moving train without any stops along the way. Skin aging in women (along with prostate health changes and male-pattern baldness) is often associated with intrinsic or chronological alterations such as hormonal changes. As previously noted, the peak of estrogen production in women occurs in their late twenties that corresponds with a peak in collagen/elastin around age 30, whereas, the continually declining trend of skin elasticity starts around 10-15 years of age (see Figure 3). Thus, the fast moving train of skin aging needs to be slowed down in order to delay the onset/development of facial wrinkles and in some cases reverse the wrinkling process to support good dermal health. What is an effective treatment for slowing down the fast moving train of facial aging? Surgery is almost always an option, but with potentially more side effects (short- and long-term), whereas, cosmecetuicals (such as sunscreens and moisturizers) may be as effective over time for many individuals and assuredly less expensive.

What Are Cosmeceuticals?

Cosmeceuticals represent the blending of cosmetics and pharmaceuticals [35]. The term cosmeceutical was first coined by Dr. Albert Kligman in 1984 to describe topical products that afford both cosmetic and therapeutic benefits [36]. These products exist on the spectrum between cosmetics, which solely adorn and beautify the skin, for example, a cosmetic claim may state: a) to decrease the appearance of wrinkles, b) reveal a more youthful appearance, c) providing invigorating or energetically healthy skin or d) brighten skin and improve skin radiance, etc., without making a biological structure/function statement or assertion. Pharmaceuticals or medications can make biological or physiological structure/function claims like: a) stimulation of collagen and elastin to decrease wrinkles, b) decreasing matrix metalloproteinases to decrease wrinkles, c) improving skin repair and wound healing or d) treat abnormal pigmentation, are just a few examples. The pharmaceutical claims, in general, are subject to safety and efficacy regulation by the U.S. Food and Drug Administration (FDA). However, the FDA does not recognize the designation "cosmeceuticals" and instead considers cosmeceutical products as cosmetics. Thus, cosmeceuticals are functional cosmetics, implying that the ingredients in such formulations come from a list of materials that are generally recognized as safe, otherwise the cosmeceutical would be classified as a drug [37]. One of the greatest sources of new cosmeceutical ingredients comes from the plant kingdom [37]. Plants are rich in antioxidants because they must survive continual ultra violet radiation exposure. Plants are also thought to be safe, which meets the FDA's criteria of substances that can be put into over-the-counter formulations. Typically, if the active ingredient is safe for oral applications, then it is assumed safe when applied topically.

Flowers, seeds, stems, leaves, roots, twigs and fruits like berries, grapes, etc. from all over the world are being incorporated into cosmeceuticals. It has been proposed that cosmeceuticals can be divided into 7 main product categories (see Table 1) [38]. In choosing an effective cosmeceutical(s) regimen it is critical to match patients and their skin problems with the appropriate products. Most patients have multiple needs, and they should be matched with products that offer active ingredients with multifactorial benefits.

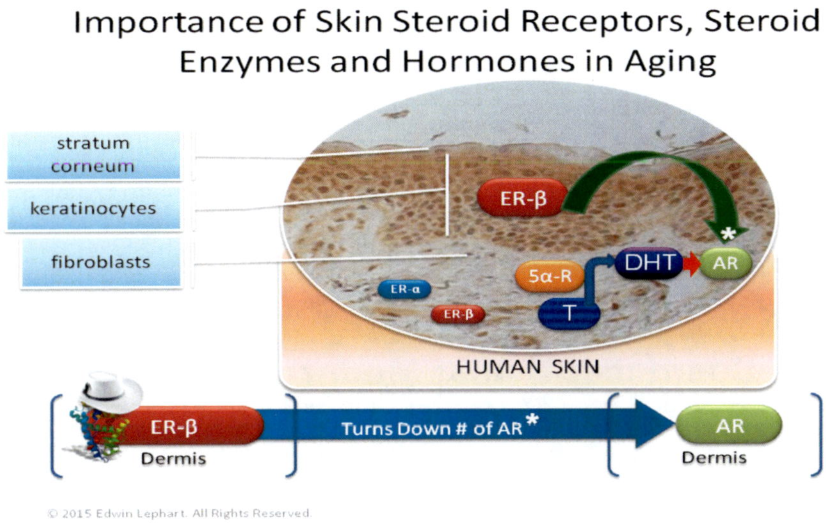

Figure 5. Steroid hormones, steroid receptors and steroid enzymes in the epidermal and dermal layers during aging. Estrogen receptor beta (ERβ), estrogen receptor alpha (ERα), androgen receptor (AR), testosterone (T), 5alpha-dihydrotestosterone (DHT), and 5alpha reductase 1 enzyme that converts testosterone to DHT in skin fibroblasts. Notably, ERα expression does not change with menopause, while ERβ expression declines by approximately 15 to 20%, thus decreasing the positive action of this estrogen receptor subtype for skin health. This is shown in the bottom portion of this figure where using a western theme, a white hat indicates activation of ERβ that is known to down-regulate the expression of androgen receptors, thus decreasing the negative impact of androgen hormone action in skin (see reference 24).

Making sure the patient is informed and using cosmeceuticals products properly is essential and some educational training may be necessary in order for each individual to receive optimal benefit [37]. For example, just think about how people diet in order to lose weight where individuals do not understand how the product/procedure works along with the importance of daily treatment/routine and more importantly daily compliance. If patients took the same approach to improve skin health then the results may be very disappointing [37]. Thus, proper understanding of the regimen, sequence or order, application volume(s), direction or pattern of applying cosmeceuticals morning and evening are critical for enhancing skin health in slowing down extrinsic and intrinsic aging.

Table 1. Cosmeceuticals product categories

1. Sunscreen
2. Anti-oxidant
3. Anti-inflammatory
4. Pigment lightening
5. Collagen repair
6. Exfoliation
7. Hydration/barrier repair

Cosmeceuticals: Modern Society's Fountain of Youth: A Snapshot of Market Shares

Like the Spanish explorer Juan Ponce de León on his mythical journey to find the fountain of youth, consumers inundated by mass media advertisements navigate aisles and counters of products purporting to slow-down, stop and/or restore skin health. Analysts report that U.S. cosmeceutical sales will top 11 billion US $ in 2016 [39] with an annual growth of 8-11% per year with L'Oreal, Proctor and Gamble, Unilever and Beiersdorf leading the way [40, 41].

The cosmeceutical markets in the U.S., the U.K., France, Germany, Italy, Spain and Japan were estimated to be worth $30.9 billion collectively in 2011, with the combined markets expected to reach $42.4 billion by 2018. The market is dominated by a small number of large players such as Procter & Gamble, L'Oreal, Unilever and Beiersdorf, who attribute their success to building big brands such as Olay, L'Oreal, Garnier and Nivea with massive marketing budgets [41]. However, other cosmetic companies with validated active ingredients provide an alternative choice for consumers.

For example, younger generations have grown up immersed in marketing messages making them both appearance-oriented and aware of the importance of preventive healthcare. As a result, new marketing prospects are opening up at the younger end of the age spectrum, even as aging "Boomers" open their wallets ever wider to stave off the cosmetic toll of aging [39]. Still, cosmeceutical marketers may take nothing for granted. Given ongoing budget constraints, shoppers expect the cosmeceuticals they buy to perform and the faster the better. Thus, any product with a quantifiable "instant gratification" benefit - has always been a powerful appeal especially in the color cosmetics category - which gives it an edge for market shares. In addition, with the upper end of the market rebounding the fastest, opportunity is greatest for premium mass-market and specialty or prestige channel products, expressing pent-up post-recession demand [39].

Cosmeceuticals are widely referred to as cosmetic products with active ingredients that have medical or drug-like benefits that patients and consumers are looking for. The difference between traditional products and the active ingredients used in topically applied cosmeceuticals really comes down to the level of biological activity within the skin, as opposed to applying a product to the skin's surface for simply an appearance benefit. However, currently there are no requirements to prove that cosmeceutical products live up to their claims [41].

While cosmeceuticals are not officially recognized by the FDA (US), cosmeceuticals must adhere to specific regulations for Good Manufacturing Practices (GMP) to ensure that products are not misbranded. Product efficacy based upon claims is scrutinized by the U.S. Federal Trade Commission (FTC), and cosmeceutical products that are perceived to be promising unrealistic expectations may be pulled from the shelves. Cosmeceutical marketers must also adhere to guidelines set by the FTC for product marketing and advertising, and face censorship for exaggerated or false product claims [41].

As consumers' technology threshold rises and they are increasingly interested in maintaining a youthful appearance, their demand for these types of high-tech products continues to expand. Yet, the more educated the consumer becomes the more important it is for the reputation of the industry to help consumers understand the term cosmeceutical, how it's used and what ways these products can be incorporated into daily routine skin care.

Botanicals (Polyphenolic Molecules) in Cosmeceuticals

Over the last decade there has been an increase in scientific interest in reducing the appearance of aging [24, 34, 42]. There are many products on the market that claim to be able to reduce aging [42, 43]. Products containing botanicals as active ingredients represent one of the largest proportion of this market [42-49]. But how does one determine if a botanical and/or cosmeceutical really does slow down skin aging?

Cosmetic approaches targeting skin aging to achieve a youthful appearance continue to emerge especially with the advancements in technology and the exchange of scientific information where physicians and patients have a greater awareness of dermal biology. Several scientific techniques have been developed. Traditional assays include cell and/or organotypic cultures to investigate the influence of a compound on human skin. Conversely, genetic strategies (gene array/mRNA levels) to identify and quantify gene expression are relatively new. Many companies only use gene expression science to make skin anti-aging claims, which makes important assumptions without validation. The best approach is to utilize both scientific tools to examine various compounds for better validation of ingredients. For example, the mechanism of action for botanicals is now beginning to be revealed both at the protein and genetic levels in describing their ameliorating roles and functions in human skin. In the following presentation these scientific approaches (both *in vitro* and *in vivo*, clinical studies) were employed to determine how effective the botanical equol that is classified as a cosmeceutical works to improve human skin anti-aging. It is important to understand how botanicals and other compounds positively influence gene expression (by stimulation or inhibition of certain genes) and compare these results to protein expression of the biomarkers. The gap can increase between chronological and biological aging where extracelluar matrix (ECM) constituents of the dermis and epidermal components are enhanced.

Equol-A Botanical with Anti-Aging Effects in Human Skin

Equol has recently caught the interest of researchers because of its powerful antioxidant activity and its unique molecular and biochemical messenger properties with implications in treating age-related diseases [50, 51]. Of particular interest, equol has an affinity for estrogen receptor beta (ER β), which is abundant in keratinocytes of the epidermis and fibroblasts in the dermis [24, 34, 52, 53].

Equol is also a selective androgen modulator (SAM), having the ability to specifically bind 5α-dihydrotestosterone (5α-DHT) and inhibit its potent negative actions in skin [24, 34, 50]. Finally, equol has the ability to bind to estrogen related receptor (ERR) gamma, which has important implications for anti-aging in human skin [34, 54, 55].

Recent evidence indicates that equol is present in plant products such as beans, cabbage, lettuces, tofu and other food products [56-59]. Equol can be found as R- and S-configuration or isomers [60-62] and the metabolism of R- and S-equol in humans appears to be similar [60, 63].

Therefore, humans are exposed to this polyphenolic compound from different plant and food sources regardless of age, gender or geographical location with scientific data to support a consumption/exposure record that appears to be safe [62-64, 65]. Moreover, equol is known to increase nuclear-factor-erythroid 2-related factor 2 (Nrf2) that plays a key role in the cellular defense against oxidative and xenobiotic stressors by its capacity to induce the expression of genes which encode detoxifying enzymes and antioxidant proteins in skin [66, 67]. Finally, equol research has dramatically increased within the past decade [61], and this polyphenolic molecule along with other botanical compounds have wide use in personal care products such as skin protectants, whitening, anti-wrinkle, and anti-aging ingredients.

Gopaul et al. [24] reported that equol has the unique characteristics to bind specifically 5α-dihydrotestosterone (5α-DHT) to decrease this negative androgen impact in skin. Equol also has affinity for estrogen receptor β (ERβ) to increase the positive estrogen-like influences in skin [24], and equol is currently used in skin treatments and positive influences on gene and protein expression (anti-aging, anti-oxidant and anti-inflammatory properties) have been reported [24].

Recently it has been proposed that ERβ agonists like S-equol may have better beneficial dermal applications [68], however, this proposition has not been confirmed by the available scientific data.

Equol: Expression of Skin-related Genes to Establish Topical Strategies that Favor Anti-oxidant, Anti-aging and Skin Regeneration

The gene (expression) array/qPCR studies where mRNA levels were quantified followed by traditional protein expression cultures using human dermal fibroblasts in short- and long-term cultures [24] are presented here for equol. From these studies, racemic equol significantly increased collagen (COL1A1), elastin (ELN), tissue inhibitor of matrix metalloproteinase 1 (TIMP 1) and significantly decreased the enzymes that breakdown collagen and elastin (the matrix metalloproteinases) or MMPs [24] (see Figure 6).

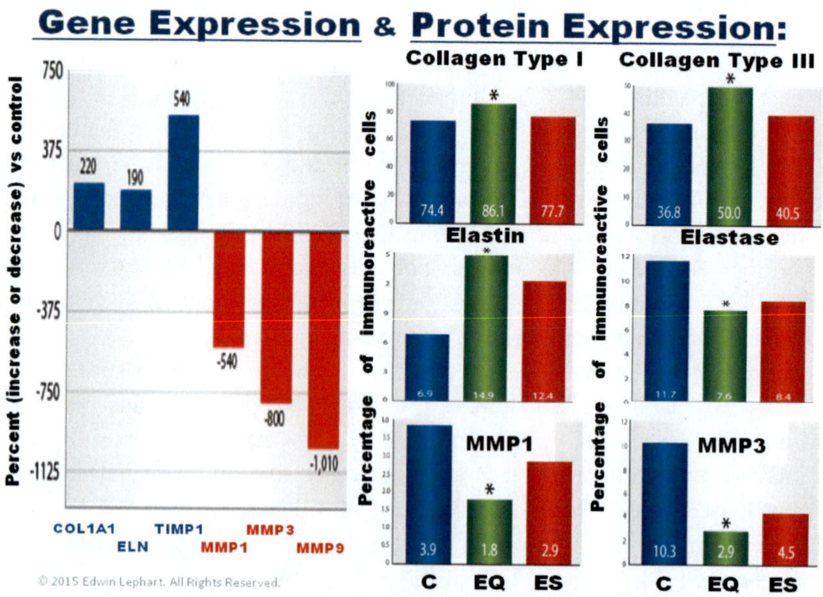

Figure 6. Validation of equol's positive influence on skin gene expression by protein expression results of various biomarkers for improved human dermal health. Gene expression was obtained by qPCR studies where mRNA levels were quantified, while protein expression was obtained from long-term (8-week) organotypic human fibroblast cultures using specific antibodies for each biomarker. In the protein expression studies 20,000 cells were quantified for each biomarker, and the percentage of immunoreactive cells are displayed by treatment: C = dimethylsulfoxide (DMSO) controls, EQ = racemic equol and ES = the natural steroid hormone, 17β-estradiol.

The y-axis range for: collagen type 1 = 0 to 100%; collagen type III = 0 to 50%; elastin = 0 to 15%; elastase = 0 to 12%; MMP1 = 0 to 4% and MMP3 = 0 to 12%. In the gene expression study, equol significantly increased collagen (COL1A1 by 220% - blue bar), elastin (ELN by 190% - blue bar), tissue inhibitor of matrix metalloproteinase 1 (TIMP 1 by 540% - blue bar), and significantly decreased the enzymes that breakdown collagen and elastin (the matrix metalloproteinases or MMPs- red bars (MMP1 by 540%, MMP3 by 800% and MMP9 by 1010%). In the long-term cultures or protein expression study, equol (green bars) significantly increased (*) collagen type I (to 86.1% •), collagen type III (to 50% or 1.4-fold higher compared to controls – blue bars, elastin (to 14.9% or 2.2-fold higher vs. controls – blue bars), and significantly decreased (*) elastase (the enzyme that breaks down elastin) to 7.6% or 1.5-fold, MMP1 to 1.8% or 2.2-fold and MMP 3 to 2.9% or 3.6-fold. In general, equol (green bars) outperformed the natural hormone, 17β-estradiol (red bars) for each quantified protein. Note•: in short-term (48-hour cultures) equol significantly increased protein expression of collagen type 1 by 1.8-fold or 180% vs. controls (DMSO), which corresponds well with the gene expression results of 220% for COL1A1 displayed here (see references 24 and 34).

However, since equol can be expressed as isomers, a recent study described a comprehensive investigation on equol as: R-equol, racemic equol or S-equol to determine their differential expression of skin-related genes and determine the percutaneous absorption in human skin using Franz cell techniques [34].

In brief, from the qPCR/mRNA studies quantifying genes expression, only three genes displayed the greatest significant expression by S-equol, whereas 16 genes displayed the greatest significant levels (either stimulation or inhibition) by R-equol and/or racemic equol, such as extracellular matrix proteins (i.e., collagen and elastin, etc.), nerve growth factor, aging genes [FOS, 100 A8 and 100 A9 calcium-binding proteins, 5α-reductase type 1, and matrix metalloproteinases (1, 3 and 9), and inflammatory genes (e.g., interleukin-1 alpha, interleukin-6, and cyclooxygenase-1) [34]. These data (in general) are summarized in Figure 7.

Additionally, the percutaneous absorption data demonstrated that equol penetrates into human skin with an unusual delivery profile [34] (see Figure 8). Notably, racemic equol is sequestered into the epidermal compartment due to the abundance of estrogen receptor subtypes in keratinocytes for which equol has a high affinity [34, 34, 52, 53, 63]. This notion is supported by quantification of the [^{3}H]-equol in the epidermis where the content was higher than typically seen with most other compounds such as other polyphenolic molecules like resveratrol along with the isoflavonoid, genistein, or topical drugs like 17β-estradiol [69-72]. The reservoir forming properties of racemic equol in the epidermis may be due to its lipophilic characteristics where its octanol-water partition coefficient is 3.20, which is higher than other polyphenolic molecules [73]. The reservoir forming properties of equol are shown in Figure 9.

Skin Antioxidant, Growth Factor, Aging and Inflammatory Biomarkers for: R-Equol, Racemic Equol and S-Equol

Gene Symbol	Gene Name	R-Equol	Racemic Equol	S-Equol
Antioxidant				
MT1H	Metallothionein-1H	2,100 + 70	2,270 + 63<	3,840 + 37<<
PCNA	Proliferating Cell Nuclear Antigen	235 + 15	285 + 11■	325 + 10■
Growth Factor				
NGF	Nerve Growth Factor	3,350 + 15>>	2,860 + 32>	1,620 + 22
Aging				
FOS	FOS (Immediate early gene)	320 + 19	340 + 9>	315 + 9
S100 A8	S100 Calcium-binding Protein A8	-2,050 + 24♦	-2,200 + 32♦♦	-580 + 28
S100 A9	S100 Calcium-binding Protein A9	-1,850 + 17♦	-2,250 + 27♦♦	-525 + 31
SRD5A1	Steroid 5α-Reductase 1	-200 + 9♣♣	-175 + 10♦	0
TNFRSF1A	Tumor Necrosis Factor Receptor 1A	-310 + 10♣♣	-250 + 19	-205 + 22
Inflammatory				
IL1A	Interleukin 1 Alpha	-1,385 + 17♦	-1,700 + 27♦♦	-990 + 42
IL1R2	Interleukin 1 Receptor 2	-1,730 + 26	-2,250 + 31♦♦	-1,675 + 45
IL6	Interleukin 6	-550 + 20♣♣	-455 + 39♦	-375 + 29
IL8	Interleukin 8	-295 + 21	-345 + 24	-445 + 33♠
PTGS1 (COX1)	Cyclooxygenase 1	-360 + 10♣♣	-265 + 25♦	-200 + 15

Figure 7. Comparison of isomers: equol (R-equol or S-equol) vs. racemic equol in the stimulation or inhibition of gene expression for skin-related biomarkers. Gene expression was quantified by qPCR/mRNA levels by Taqman florescence detection. Each Gene Symbol/Name is color-coded indicating the equol form with the greatest (stimulation or inhibition) expression level.
< Significantly greater stimulation compared to R-equol; << Significantly greater stimulation compared to Racemic equol or R-equol; > Significantly greater stimulation compared to S-equol; >> Significantly greater stimulation compared to Racemic equol or S-equol; ■ Significantly greater stimulation compared to R-equol; ♦ Significantly greater inhibition compared to S-equol; ♦♦ Significantly greater inhibition compared to R-equol or S-equol; ♣♣ Significantly greater inhibition compared to Racemic equol or S-equol; ♠ Significantly greater inhibition compared to Racemic equol or R-equol. 1.2% equol (treatments: R-equol, Racemic equol or S-equol) in DMSO vehicle vs. DMSO control levels; n = 6. Values represent percentage (%) increase or decrease vs. control values, followed by pairwise comparisons among treatment groups (mean + SEM) of gene array analysis, p < 0.005 for all data (see reference 34).

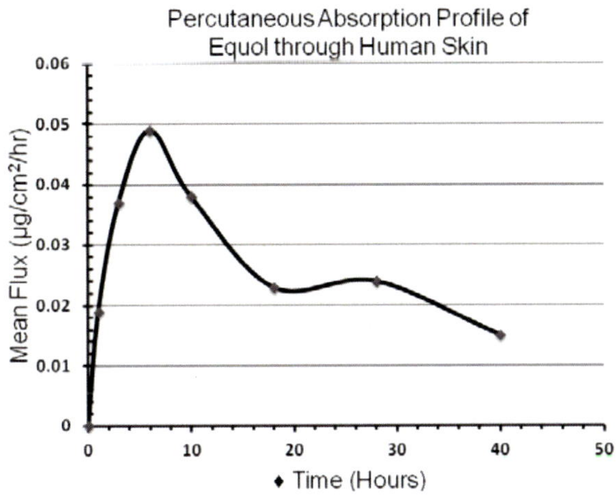

Figure 8. [^{3}H]-Equol Percutaneous Absorption Profile into Human Skin
[^{3}H]-equol was used to determine percutaneous absorption into human skin with a profile showing an initial maximum peak flux occurring 6 h after dosing followed by a decline with a secondary lower peak at approximately 26-28 h after a single applied dose. Human trunk skin obtained from 4 individuals (2 males and 2 females of Caucasian and Hispanic decent, ages 35 to 51, n = 3 per subject) were tested by Franz cell techniques. The standard error of the mean (SEM) among the time point collections ranged from 0.005 to 0.024 (not shown graphically). (see reference 34)

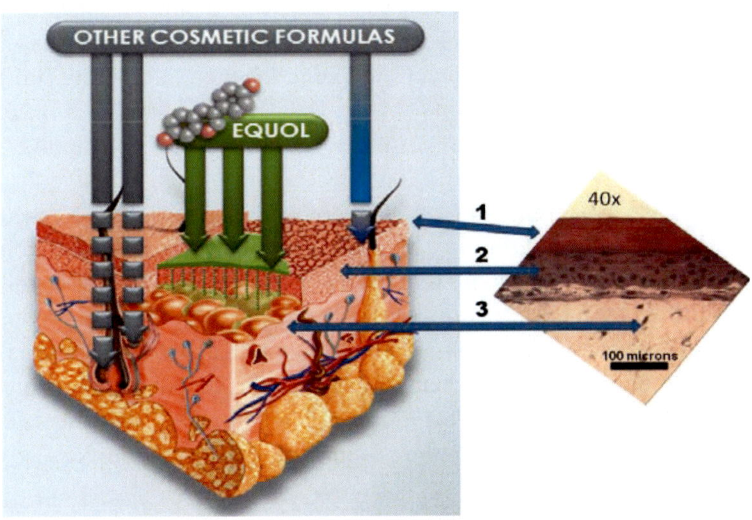

Figure 9. Cartoon display of typical active ingredients versus equol in penetrating human skin layers (left panel).

Histological magnification (40 x) of epidermal and dermal human skin layers (right panel). Almost all typical cosmetic/cosmeceutical ingredients either do not penetrate the human skin layers at all or pass through the skin layers with a typical bell-shaped profile with a short duration (left panel, blue or gray arrows). Remarkably, equol is sequestered into the epidermal compartment due to its affinity to and the abundance of estrogen receptor subtypes in keratinocytes (green arrows) and forms an equol reservoir that has a time-release prolife into the dermis to act upon fibroblasts and promote anti-aging effects in human skin. 1 = stratum coreum and 2 = keratinocytes (in the epidermis); 3 = fibroblasts in the dermis.

Finally, when the above equol skin biomarker results are compared to the botanical that has the highest recognized general public or lay profile namely, resveratrol [74], equol universally displayed better biochemical, molecular, protective and delivery mechanisms of action to promote improve human skin health as a topical anti-aging ingredient/compound.

Conclusion

It is important to understand the characteristics of skin aging and the concept and use of cosmeceuticals in slowing down the aging process. Notably, botanicals, as active ingredients, represent one of the largest percentages of compounds in use in cosmeceuticals today. A botanical with superior promise for human skin anti-aging is the isoflavonoid molecule, equol based upon its molecular weight, lipophilic nature and ability to bind specifically to the potent androgen, 5α-DHT to decrease this negative hormonal impact in skin. Equol also has positive actions to improve skin health by its ability to bind to ERβ and ERR gamma in human skin that are abundant in the epidermis and fibroblasts found in the dermis. Moreover, equol can activate Nrf2 to defend against oxidative stress and increase detoxifying enzymes and antioxidants. In examining the isomers of equol, the results illustrate the significant differences in mirror-image molecules of equol for skin-related gene and protein expression that clearly demonstrate: a) R-equol and/or racemic equol are better molecules for dermal gene and protein expression in anti-aging effects compared to S-equol and b) the percutaneous absorption of racemic equol represents an unique epidermal reservoir delivery mechanism.

References

[1] Klaassen, CD. Ed. Casarett and Doull's Toxicology: The Basic Science of Poisions. 5th ed. New York, N.Y. McGraw-Hill, 1996, 529-546.

[2] Qunshan, J; J Frank Nash. Pathology of Aging Skin, In: Textbook of Aging Skin, Eds. MA Farage, KW Miller, HI Maibach, Springer-Verlag, Berlin Heidelberg, 2010, 277-291.

[3] Madison, KC. Barrier function of the skin: "la raison d'etre" of the epidermis, *J Invest Dermatol*, 2003, 121, 231-241.

[4] Menon, GK. New insights into skin structure: scratching the surface. *Adv Drug Delivery Rev*, 2002, 54, S3-S17.

[5] Farage, MA; Miller, KW; Maibach HI. Degenerative Changes in Aging Skin, In: Textbook of Aging Skin, Eds. MA Farage, KW Miller, HI Maibach, Springer-Verlag, Berlin Heidelberg, 2010, 225-35.

[6] Brincat, MP, Baron, YM, Galea, R. Estrogens and the skin. *Climacteric*, 2005, 8, 110-123.

[7] Lephart, ED. Review Human Biology, Dubuque Iowa, Kendall/Hunt, 2009, 77-78.

[8] Pierard, GE; Paquet, P; Xhauflaire-Uhoda, E; Quatresooz, P. Physiological Variations During Aging, In: Textbook of Aging Skin, Eds. MA Farage, KW Miller, HI Maibach, Springer-Verlag, Berlin Heidelberg, 2010, 45-54.

[9] Martini, F. Fundamentals of anatomy and physiology. San Francisco, CA, Benjamin-Cummings, 2004.

[10] US Bureau of the Census. *An Aging World*. 2004.

[11] Farage, MA; Miller, KW; Elsener, P; et al. Intrinsic and extrinsic factors in skin aging: a review. *Internat J Cosmetic Sci*, 2008, 30, 87-95.

[12] Friedman, O. Changes associated with the aging face, *Facial Plast Surg Clin North Am*, 2005, 13, 371-380.

[13] Duncan, KO; Leffell, DJ. Preoperative assessment of the elderly patient, *Dermatol Clin*, 1997, 15, 583-593.

[14] Kligman, AM; Koblenzer, C. Demographics and psychological implications for the aging population, *Dermtol Clin*, 1997, 15, 549-553.

[15] Glogua, RG. Systemic evaluation of the aging face. In: Dermatology, Eds. Bolognia, JL, Jorizzo, JL, Rapini, RP, Mosby, Edinburgh, 2003.

[16] Badia, AA. Skin Aging-Clincial Evaluation & Treatment of Aging Skin, In: Encyclopedia of Clinical Anti-Aging Medicine & Regenerative Biomedical Technologies, Eds. Klatz, R & Goldman, R, The American Academy of Anti-Aging Medicine, Chicago, IL, 609-639.

[17] Khol, E; Steinbauer, J; Landthaler, M; Szeimies, RM. Skin Aging, *J European Acad Dermatol Venereol*, 2011, 25, 873-884.
[18] Freedberg, IM; Eisen, AZ; Wolff, K; Austen, KF; Goldsmith, LA; Katz, SI. Fritzpatrick's Dermatology in General Medicine, 6th ed, McGraw Hill, 2003.
[19] Burns, DA; Breathnach, SM. Rook's Textbook of Dermatology, 7th ed, Blackwell Publishing Co, Vol 1, 3.1 and 4.1, 2004.
[20] Baumann, L. Cosmetic Dermatology: Principles and Practice, McGraw Hill, Hong Kong, 2002.
[21] Schwartz, D, Mayaux, MJ. Female fecundity as a function of age: results of artificial insemination in 2193 nulliparous women with azoospermic husbands. *New England J Med*, 1982, 306, 404-406.
[22] Jain, T; Klein, NA; Lee, DM; Sluss, PM; Soules, MR. Endocrine assessment of relative reproductive age in normal eumenorrheic younger and older women across multiple cycles. *Am J Obstet Gynecol*, 2003, 189, 1080-1084.
[23] Escoffier, C; de Rigal, J; Rachdfore, A; Vasselet, R; Lefeque, JL; Agache, PG. Age-related mechanical properties of human skin: an in vivo study. *J Invest Dermatol*, 1989, 93, 353-357.
[24] Gopaul, R; Knaggs, H; Lephart, ED. Biochemical investigation and gene analysis of equol: A plant and soy-derived isoflavonoid with anti-aging and anti-oxidant properties with potential human skin applications, *Biofactors*, 2012, 38, 44-52.
[25] Hillebrand, GG. Facial Wrinkling: The Marquee Clinical Sign of Aging Skin, In: Textbook of Aging Skin, Eds. MA Farage, KW Miller, HI Maibach, Springer-Verlag, Berlin Heidelberg, 2010, 911-918.
[26] Uitto, J. The role of elastin and collagen in cutaneous aging: intrinsic aging versus photoexposure. *J Drugs Dermatol*, 2008, 7, S12-S16.
[27] Fujimura, T; Haketa, K; Hotta, M; Kitahara, T. Loss of skin elasticity precedes to rapid increase of wrinkle levels. *J Dermatol Sci*, 2007, 47, 233-239.
[28] Hillebrand, GG; Levine, MJ; Miyamoto, K. The age-dependent changes in skin condition in African Americans, Caucasians, East Asians, Indian Asians and Latinos, *IFSCC Mag*, 2001, 4, 259-266.
[29] Miyamoto, K; Hillebrand, GG. The influence of facial expression on the age-dependent changes in facial wrinkling, *J Soc Cos Sci*, 2007, 58, 206-2007.

[30] Hillebrand, GG; Yoshii, T; Yan, X. Progession of temporary into persistent facial wrinkling: An 8-year longitudinal study, *J Am Acad Derm*, 2009, 60, AB1.

[31] Akazaki, S; Nakagawa, H; Kazama, H. Age-related changes in skin wrinkles assessed by a novel three-dimensional morphometric analysis, *Br J Dermatol*, 2002, 147, 689-695.

[32] Kuwazuru, O; Saothong, J; Yoshikawa, Y. Mechanical approach to aging and wrinkling of human facial skin based on the multistage buckling theory, *Med Eng Phys*, 2008, 30, 516-522.

[33] Phillips, TJ; Symons, J; Menon, S. HT Study Group. Does hormone therapy improve age-related skin changes in postmenopausal women? *J Am Acad Derm*atol, 2008, 59, 397-404.

[34] Lephart, ED. Protective effects of equol and their polyphenolic isomers against dermal aging: Microarray/protein evidence with clinical implications and unique delivery into human skin, *Pharmaceutical Biol*, 2013, 51, 1391-1400.

[35] Green, JB; Metelitsa, AI. *Introduction, Seminars in Cutaneous Medicine Surgery*, 2011, 30, 1-2.

[36] Kligman, A. The future of cosmeceuticals: An interview with Albert Kligman, MD, PhD. Interviewed by Dr. Zoe Diana Draelos, *Dermatol Surg*, 2005, 31, 890-981.

[37] Draelos, ZD. The Art and Science of New Advances in Cosmeceuticals, *Clin Plastic Surg*, 2011, 38, 397-407.

[38] Reszko, A; Berson, D; Lupo, MP. Cosmeceuticals: Practical Applications, *Obstet Gynecol Clin North Am*, 2010, 37, 547-569.

[39] The US: Cosmeceutical Market @ http://www.prnewswire.com/news-releases/cosmeceuticals-in-the-us-6th-edition-161782015.html

[40] Cosmeceutical Skincare Production Market Research Report/Life Sciences/Wellness Nutrition and Supplements, January 2013, IBISWorld's Cosmeceutical Skincare Production market research report.

[41] Cosmeceuticals Market to 2018-Technological Advances and Consumer Awareness Boost Commerical Potential for Innovative and Premium-priced Products, New Research Says Cosmeceuticals Rank as the Fastest Growing Beauty Category, January 31, 2013 by GBI Research http://www.gcimagazine.com/marketstrends/segments/antiaging/New-Research-Says-Cosmeceuticals-Rank-as-the-Fastest-Growing-Beauty-Category-189246721.html

[42] Hunt, KJ; Hung, SK; Ernst, E. Botanical Extracts as Anti-aging Preparations for the Skin, *Drugs Aging*, 2010, 27, 973-985.

[43] Perls, TT. Hope Drives Anti-aging Hype, *Cleveland Clin J Med*, 2006, 73, 1039-1044.

[44] Thornefeldt, C. Cosmeceuticals Containing Herbs: Fact, Fiction and Future, *Dermatol Surg*, 2005, 37, 873-880.

[45] Baumann, LS. Less-known Cosmeceuticals, *Dermatol Ther*, 2007, 20, 339-342.

[46] Bogdan, Allemann I; Baumann, L. Antioxidants used in skincare formulations, *Skin Ther Lett*, 2008, 13, 1-12.

[47] Chiu, A; Kimball, AB. Topical Vitamins, Minerals and Botanical Ingredients as Modulators or Environmental and Chronological Skin Damage, *Br J Dermatol*, 2003, 149, 681-691.

[48] Cronin, H; Draelos, ZD. Top 10 Botanical Ingredients in 2010 anti-aging creams, *J Cosmetic Dermatology*, 2010, 9, 218-225.

[49] Gao, XH; Zhang, L; Wei, H. Efficacy and Safety of Innovative Cosmeceuticals, *Clin Dermatol*, 2008, 26, 367-374.

[50] Lund, TD; Blake, C; Bu, L; Hamaker, AN; Lephart, ED. Equol an isoflavonoid: potential for improved prostate health, in vitro and in vivo evidence. *Reprod Biol Endocrinol*, 2011, 9, 4.

[51] Blake, C; Fabick, KM; Setchell, KDR; Lund, TD; Lephart, ED. Neuromodulation by Soy Diet or Equol: Anti-depressive & Anti-obesity-like Influences, Age- & Hormone-dependent Effects. *BMC Neuroscience*, 2011, 12, 8.

[52] Thornton, MJ; Taylor, AH; Mulligan, K; Al-Azzawi, F; Lyon, CC; O'Driscoll, J. Messenger, AG. Oestrogen receptor beta is the predominant oestrogen receptor in human scalp skin, *Exper Dermatol*, 2003, 12, 181-190.

[53] Pelletier, G; Ren, L. Localization of sex steroid receptors in human skin, *Histology and Histopathology*, 2004, 19, 629-636.

[54] Hirvonen, J; Rajalin, AM; Wohlfart, G; Adlercreutz, H; Wähälä, K; Aarnisalo, P. Transcriptional activation of estrogen-related receptor gamma (ERRgamma) is stimulated by the phytoestrogen equol. *J Steroid Biochem Mole Biol*, 2011, 123, 46-57.

[55] Krahn-Bertil, E; Bolzinger, MA; Andre, V; Orly, I; Kanitakis, J; Rousselle, P; Damour, O. Expression of estrogen-related receptor gamma (ERRgamma) in human skin. *Eur J Dermatol*, 2008, 18, 427-432.

[56] Hounsome, N; Hounsome, B; Deri Tomos, A; Edwards-Jones, G. Changes in anti-oxidant compounds in white cabbage during winter storage. *Postharvest Biol Tech*, 2009, 52, 173-179.

[57] Hounsome, N; Grail, B; Deri Tomos, A; Hounsome, B; Edwards-Jones, G. High-throughput anti-oxidant profiling in vegetables by Fourier-transform ion Cyclotron resonance mass spectrometry. *Functional Plant Sci Biotech*, 2010, 4, 1-10.

[58] Abiru, Y; Kumenura, M; Ueno, T; Uchiyama, S; Masaki, K. Discovery of an S-equol rich food stinky tofu, a traditional fermented soy product in Taiwan, *Internat J Food Sci Nutr*, 2012, 63, 964-970.

[59] Jou, H-J; Tsai, P-J; Tu, J-H; Wu, W-H. Stinky tofu as a rich source of biavailable S-equol in Asian diets, *J Functional Foods*, 2013, 5, 651-659.

[60] Setchell, KDR; Clerici, C; Lephart, ED; Cole, SJ; Heenan, C; Heenan, C; Castellani, D; Wolfe, BE; Nechemias-Zimmer, L; Brown, NM; Lund, TD; Handa, RJ. S-Equol, a potent ligand for estrogen receptor {beta}, is the exclusive enantiomeric form of the soy isoflavone metabolite produced by human intestinal bacterial flora. *Am J Clin Nutr*, 2005, 81, 1072-1079.

[61] Setchell, KDR; Clerici, C. Equol: History, Chemistry, and Formation. *J Nutr*, 2010, 140, 1355S-1362S.

[62] Lephart, ED. Chapter 29. Isoflavones and Prenatal Exposure to Equol. In Isoflavones: Chemistry, Analysis, Function and Effects (V.R. Preedy, ed.), The Royal Society of Chemistry, Thomas Graham House, Cambridge, England, United Kingdom, 2013, 480-499.

[63] Setchell, KDR; Zhao, X; Jah, P; Heubi, JE; Brown, NM. The pharmacokinetic behavior of the soy isoflavone metabolite S-(-) equol and its diastereoisomer R-(+)equol in healthy adults determined by using stable-isotope-labeled tracers. *Am J Clin Nutr*, 2009, 90, 1029-1037.

[64] Frankenfeld, CL. Dairy consumption is a significant correlate of urinary equol concentration in representative sample of US adults. *Am J Clin Nutr*, 2011, 93, 1109-1116.

[65] Munro, IC; Harwood, M; Hlywka, JJ; Stephen, AM; Doull, JD; Flamm, WG; Adlercreutz, H. Soy Isoflavones: A Safety Review. *Nutr Rev*, 2003, 61, 1-33.

[66] Zhang, T; Xinyu, L; Shi, L; Wang, L; Chen, J; Kang, C; Zhu, J; Mi, M. Estrogen receptor and PI3K/Akt signaling pathway involvement in S-(-) equol-induced activation of Nrf2/ARE in endothelial cells. *Plos One*, 2013, 8, e79075.

[67] Beyer, TA; Keller, U; Braun, S; Schafer, M; Werner, S. Roles and mechanisms of action of the Nrf2 transcription factor in skin

morphogenesis, wound repair and skin cancer. *Cell Death Differentiation*, 2007, 14, 1250-1254.

[68] Jackson, RL; Greiwe, JS; Schwen, RJ. Ageing skin: Oestrogen receptor beta agonists offer an approach to change the outcome. *Exp Dermatol,* 2011, 20, 879-882.

[69] Chadha, G; Sathigari, S; Parsons, DL; Jayachandra, BR. In vitro percutaneous absorption of genistein from topical gels through human skin. *Drug Dev Indust Pharm*, 2011, 37, 498-505.

[70] Hung, C-F; Lin, Y-K; Huang, Z-R; Fang, JY. Delivery of resveratrol, a red wine polyphenol, for solutions and hydrogels via the skin, *Bio Pharm Bull*, 2008, 31, 955-962.

[71] Xing, MH; Hui, X; Zhong, W. In vitro human topical bioactive drug transdermal absorption: Estradiol, *Cutanenous Ocular Toxicol*, 2009, 28, 171-175.

[72] Zhong, W; Xing, MMQ; Hui, X; Maibach, HI A stochastic model for transepidermal drug delivery. *Skin Res Tech*, 2009, 15, 407-411.

[73] Rothwell, JA; Day, AJ; Morgan, MR. Experimental determination of octanol-water partition coefficients of quercetin and related flavonoids. *J Agr Food Chem*, 2005, 53, 4355-4360.

[74] Lephart, ED; Summerfeldt, JM; Andrus, MB. Resveratrol: Influences on gene expression in human skin. *J Functional Foods*, 2014. 10, 377-384.

In: Skin Aging and Photoaging
Editor: Emanuel Graham
ISBN: 978-1-63482-907-6

Chapter 3

New Insights on the Role of Pollution in Regulation of Skin Physiology and Aging

Simarna Kaur, Michelle Garay, Marisa Dufort and Michael D. Southall*

Johnson & Johnson Skin Research Center, CPPW, a Division of Johnson & Johnson Consumer Companies, Inc. Skillman, New Jersey, US

Abstract

Our skin is under continuous assault from a variety of damaging environmental factors including ultraviolet irradiation and atmospheric pollutants such as smoke and ozone, and environmental aggression such as heat and cold temperatures. Extrinsic factors, particularly sunlight, have been demonstrated to accelerate the intrinsic aging process, resulting in elastosis, inflammation, and increased matrix protein degradation. Other factors such as chronic smoke exposure have been shown to affect skin aging; however few studies have ever examined the holistic effects of the cumulative exposure to pollution and external aggression. On a daily basis, the skin is exposed to a variety of environmental aggressors including solar UV radiation and atmospheric pollutants. This exposure

* Corresponding author: Dr. Michael Southall, Johnson & Johnson Consumer Companies, Inc., 199 Grandview Road, Skillman, NJ 08558, Phone: 908-874-2318 ; Fax: 908-874-1209, Email: msoutha@its.jnj.com.

can result in harmful effects on skin health. The chapter will report on the types of pollution and external aggression that skin is exposed to, and will review recent published studies that report that cumulative exposure to five daily environmental aggressors (pollution, sun, cold, heat and wind) synergistically increase this skin damage. Measures of oxidative damage, cytokine levels and cell viability will be discussed and the effects of increased production of ROS and inflammatory cytokines, after exposure to each of the environmental stressors (UV radiation, ozone, excessive heat and humidity, cigarette smoke, and cold wind) will be examined. A number of skin care product ingredients will be reviewed which have scientific data to suggest they may provide protection or repair from the skin damaging effect of pollution. The mechanisms of action for these ingredients will be reviewed along with specific examples of how they manifest skin protection from pollution. Finally the chapter will discuss clinical studies of topical formulations reported to protect skin from pollution. For example in one study topical application of a cream containing anti-pollution actives significantly decreased the production of ROS, inflammatory cytokines, and mitochondrial damage induced by a combination of UV and pollution. Taken together, the chapter will review literature and present data demonstrating that the cumulative effect of exposing skin to everyday pollution can affect skin physiology, alter the skin barrier and may accelerate the skin aging process.

Introduction

Skin under External Aggression and Inflammation

Our skin is first barrier between our bodies and the environment, providing protection from the environment's chemical and physical challenges. Depending on geographic location and lifestyle choices external factors such as ultraviolet radiation, extreme hot and cold temperatures, variable humidity, and air pollution impose constant challenges to the skin barrier and can contribute to skin aging. To function effectively the skin must be resilient in overcoming the detrimental effects of these assaults. Generally, environmental stressors result in formation of oxidative compounds, eventually leading to oxidative stress, inflammation, and cellular damage, all of which ultimately contribute to degradation of skin matrix proteins which manifests as signs of skin aging, such as wrinkles. Additionally, exposure of the skin to air pollutants has also been associated with allergic skin conditions such as atopic dermatitis, eczema, psoriasis or acne, while skin cancer is among the most serious effects [1]

Intrinsic aging, linked to genetic factors, is an inevitable fate for all skin, with visible manifestations including loss of elasticity, and thinning skin with exaggerated expression lines. However, it is widely accepted that extrinsic, external aggression-induced aging, characterized by coarse wrinkles, and pigmented lesions accounts for the majority of the visible signs of skin aging. Indeed between 40%-90% of the aged appearance of the skin is attributed to extrinsic aging [2, 3]. To isolate the effects of extrinsic skin aging, Guyuron et al. studied the effect of UV exposure and cigarette smoke on the apparent age of identical twins [4]. The researchers showed that higher apparent age correlated with increased outdoor activity, and cigarette smoke. They also demonstrated an increased aged appearance for participants who used less sunscreen.

Several lines of evidence suggest that extrinsic aging is mediated by inflammation. Inflammation is the natural protective mechanism to correcting physiological challenges such as infection, DNA damage, and wound repair. However, due to the destructive nature of inflammation, protection comes at the cost of tissue damage. An initial step in translating environmental signals to inflammation is through the formation of highly reactive oxidative compounds. Though extremely short-lived, these reactive oxygen species (ROS) can confer direct damage to tissues. Furthermore, these compounds may be quasi-stabilized by formation of secondary oxidative molecules such as lipid peroxides, which may diffuse to surrounding tissues, resulting in deeper inflammatory tissue damage. To some extent, the skin is equipped with a biochemical system of antioxidant release pathways that offset oxidative damage. However, chronic exposure leads to accumulation of these oxidants and eventually overwhelms endogenous antioxidant supplies, leading to oxidative stress, and inflammation. Consequently, the onset of inflammation promotes additional generation of oxidative compounds as well as enzymes that degrade the skin matrix proteins (e.g., matrix metalloproteinases, MMP). As such, an inflammatory response arising from environmental exposure may lead to a vicious cycle that amplifies the effects of the environment on tissue damage and skin aging.

The most significant environmental challenges, with respect to skin aging, are from UV radiation, by way of sun exposure, and air pollution, including exposure to cigarette smoke. Chronic exposure to these factors has been shown to result in cumulative damage to skin constituents, leading to premature skin thinning, wrinkling, and hyperpigmentation which contribute to the aged appearance of the skin [5, 6, 7]. There are reduced levels of extracellular matrix proteins, such as collagen and elastin, in aged skin. Additionally, there is a diminished capacity to regenerate ECM proteins in aged skin, magnifying the effect of inflammation on skin aging for older individuals.

Below are reviewed the effects of various environmental stressors, all of which may lead to oxidative stress, inflammation, and MMP release, ultimately resulting in diminished extracellular matrix protein constituents, which is a primary cause of aged appearance of skin. This is the currently accepted central paradigm of extrinsic skin aging.

UV Exposure and Skin Inflammation

It is widely accepted that cumulative UV exposure is the major cause of premature skin aging in today's middle aged and elderly population, leading to so-called photoaging, ultimately by means of damage to the skin's connective tissue. The relatively recent depletion of the protective stratospheric ozone layer increases the susceptibility of the skin to UV damage. The subset of UV radiation involved in skin aging is broken into two classifications, each with varying biochemical effects. The higher energy UV-B (280-315 nm) affects the outermost layer of the skin, whereas the lower energy UV-A (315-400 nm) penetrates beyond the epidermis.

Kligman et al., demonstrated elastic fiber damage and dermal tissue hypertrophy following either UVA or UVB exposure [8]. They also demonstrated summation of the deleterious effects when co-administered. As solar radiation inseparably contains UVA and UVB, this work highlights the need for photoprotection against both bands to prevent damaging effects of UV (broad spectrum protection).

Ultraviolet radiation elicits tissue and cellular damage either directly via immediate interaction between photons and skin constituents, or indirectly, through generation of reactive oxygen species (ROS). Direct UV damage may occur via cyclobutane-pyrimidine dimerization (CPD), leading to mutations during DNA replication. Direct photoreaction also results in formation of the most common DNA lesion, 8-oxo-guanine, causing mismatched replication and mutation. Indirect effects of UV result from the oxidative action of UV induced ROS on various skin constituents, including DNA, proteins, and lipids.

Whether by direct or indirect mechanisms, UV exposure induces inflammatory responses in the skin, leading to the release of ECM-degrading MMPs. It has been shown that even very low doses of UV radiation up-regulate AP-1 and NF-kB (Nuclear Factor Kappa-light-chain-enhancer of activated B cells) DNA binding, leading to induction of the MMPs, collagenase, 92-kd gelatinase, and stromelysin-1. Additionally UV exposure has been shown to increase MMP-3, MMP-9, and MMP-12 [9, 10]. Fisher et al., showed that controlled UV exposure of non-exposed skin resulted in 58% greater degradation of type I collagen fibrils compared to non-irradiated control skin in vivo [11]. Prolonged activity of MMPs in the skin leads to abnormal rates of dermal degradation of collagen and elastin which lead to premature aging.

Environmental Pollution and Skin Inflammation

Rapid industrialization has led to increased levels of environmental air pollution, particularly in highly populated metropolitan cities. Consequently, populations living in highly industrialized areas have been linked to having a higher incidence of certain health conditions such as cancer, and pulmonary and cardiovascular diseases. Air pollution has also been implicated in accelerating skin aging due to the pro-oxidant and pro-inflammatory nature of air pollutants.

Particulate Matter

Particulate matter (PM) is one such air pollutant. Characterized as nanoparticulate matter suspended in the air, such as those originating from fossil fuel combustion, cigarette smoke, or industrial processes, PM's are a growing concern with potential to affect millions worldwide. In addition to their own inherent toxicity, PM's act as carriers for other detrimental environmental agents such as polycyclic aromatic hydrocarbons (PAH) and metals [12]. Due to their small size PMs penetrate into the skin and co-deliver adsorbed toxic agents [13]. Polycyclic aromatic hydrocarbons such as benzo[a]pyrene (BaP) can be found in the air, food, and water as a result of incomplete combustion of fossil fuels (from power plants, car exhaust, heaters, and cigarette smoke) [14]. Particulate matter has been postulated to induce ROS in skin [15]. Li et al., suggested that these particles may enter the mitochondria and initiate ROS generation [12]. Studies have not yet directly connected skin exposure to particulate matter and MMP release. However, it has been shown that metal nanoparticles do upregulate MMP-2, and MMP-9 induction in monocytes, via ROS generation [16]. Vierkotter et al., investigated the clinical influence of PM levels on inflammation and aging in 400 Caucasian women, indicating a correlation between a composite aging score and local particulate matter levels [17].

Tobacco Smoke

Given that smoking tobacco products is strongly associated with many diseases including lung cancer, emphysema, and cardiovascular disease, it comes as no surprise that smokers physically appear older than their true age. Cigarette smoke has been associated with premature skin aging since the mid-1800s [18]. Oxidative compounds in cigarette smoke generate ROS upon exposure to lung and skin tissues. Similar to UV exposure, cigarette smoke initiates a cascade of events leading to inflammation, MMP release, and premature aging [19].

Cigarette smoke induces significantly greater MMP-1 gene expression in skin of smokers compared to non-smokers, implying systemic inflammatory effects of smoking [20]. Yin et al., demonstrated increased MMP3 mRNA in human fibroblasts following exposure to the water soluble fraction of tobacco smoke [21]. In addition, they showed that collagen biosynthesis was reduced by 40%. On the other hand, tissue inhibitors of matrix metalloproteinases (TIMP) were unaffected by exposure. The work exemplifies that smoking creates an imbalance of ECM processes detrimental to dermal collagen levels. Furthermore, a case study of identical twin sisters with similar lifestyle factors showed dramatic differences in severity of skin aging for the smoking twin compared to a non-smoking sister demonstrating the clinical relevance of the effects of smoke exposure [22].

As depicted in figure 1(a-b), in-vitro studies have shown that a combination of smoke and UV exposure potentiated the skin damage as measured by increases in ROS and membrane damage marker LDH.

Ozone

Ozone is the major oxidative component of photochemical smog. It is known to rapidly degrade antioxidants, induce ROS [23] and initiate inflammation in exposed tissues, including respiratory epithelia and skin. Mice exposed to ozone levels comparable to levels observed in polluted cities exhibited increased lipid peroxidation, and increased MMP-9 expression and activity, in exposed skin [24]. Human keratinocytes exposed to ozone demonstrate elevated levels of IL-1α, hydrogen peroxide, and increased DNA damage, potentially via a decrease in the NAD-dependent histone deacetylase, Sirtuin 3 [25]. Additionally, ozone has also been shown to induce the expression of cytochrome P450 genes via increased nuclear translocation of the aryl hydrocarbon receptor (AhR) [26].

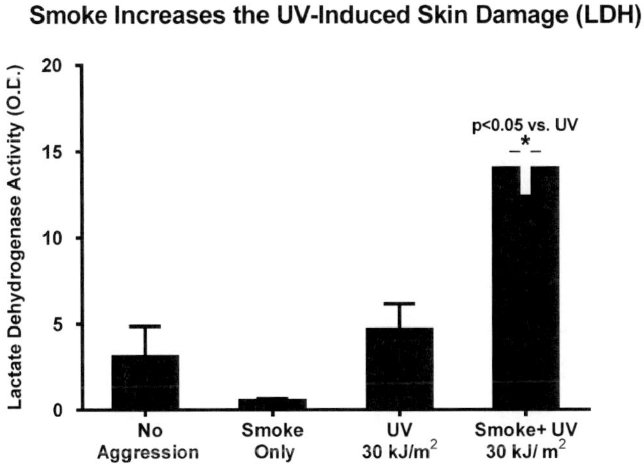

Figure 1a. I posure to cigarette smol r 30 minutes increased the UV-induced skin damage as i easured by the productic LDH (lactate dehydrogenase), a marker of membrane mage and toxicity in a human epidermal equivalent tissue model by 3-fold compared to the comparable dose of UV alone.

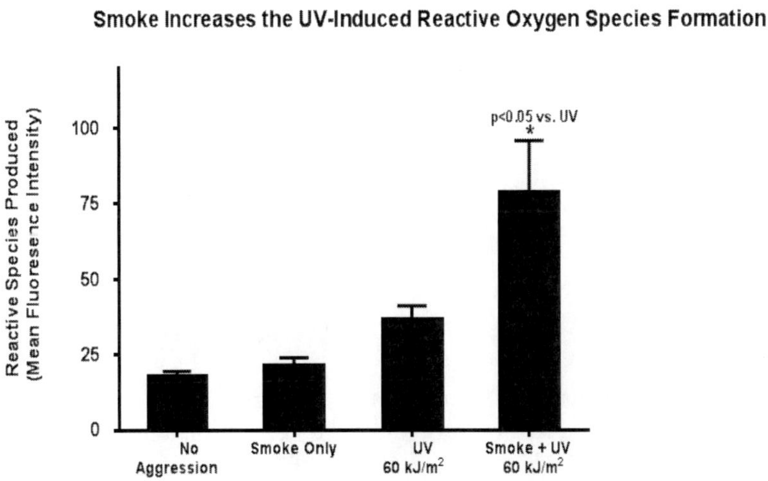

Figure 1b. The combination of Smoke and UV doubled the skin damage as measured by ROS production relative to UV alone. Exposure to cigarette smoke for 30 minutes increased the UV-induced Reactive Oxygen Species production in a human epidermal equivalent tissue model by 2-fold compared to the identical dose of UV alone.

Other Stressors

Exposure to extreme climate changes including cold, heat, and humidity can have acute or chronic effects on skin, especially in combination with UV. These climate conditions have been shown to reduce the hydration status of the epidermis and compromise the skin barrier function [27]. Furthermore, as depicted in Figure 2 below, exposing skin cells to heat or cold temperatures potentiated lipid peroxidation damage induced by UV light.'

Cold and Heat Stress Exacerbates the Oxidative Damage Caused by UV

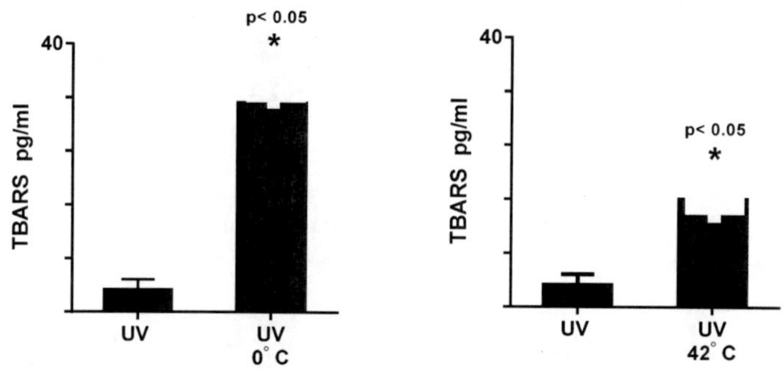

Figure 2. In cu...ured huma.. keratinocytes, oxidative damage as m..as..red by lipid peroxidation (TBARS) increased when UV-exposure was combined with cold or heat shock. Cold or Heat alone did not significant changes in lipid peroxidation.

Cumulative Effects of Multiple Environmental Stressors on Skin Can Lead to Synergistic Damage

It has been previously documented that the impact of chemical pollutants (such as BaP) which exist at levels below the toxic or tumorigenic threshold, when combined with UV, can be synergistic [14]. Along similar lines, figure 3 (a-b) below shows that the cumulative exposure to environmental stressors (UV, ozone, smoke, heat/humidity) can double the levels of pro-inflammatory cytokines as compared to UV alone indicating a synergy in the damage produced by all the stressors combined.

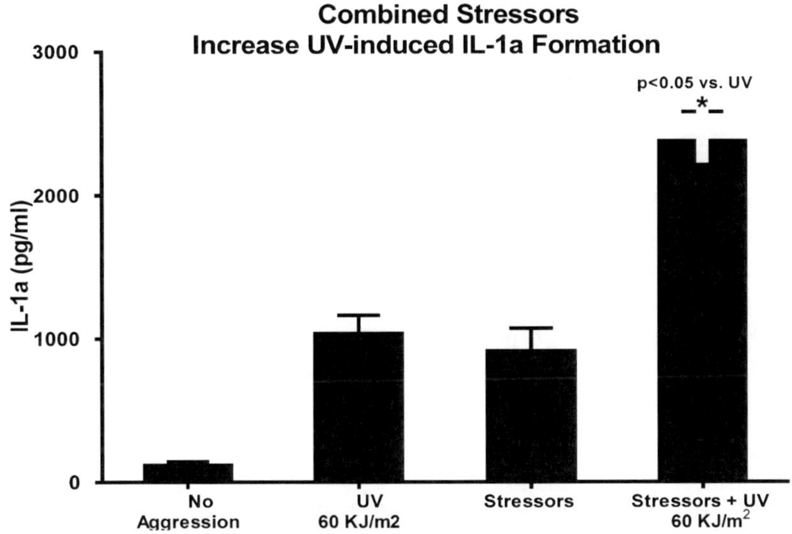

Figure 3a. Synergistic induction of pro-inflammatory marker, IL-1α, in response to the combined environmental stressors: UV, ozone, smoke, heat/humidity.

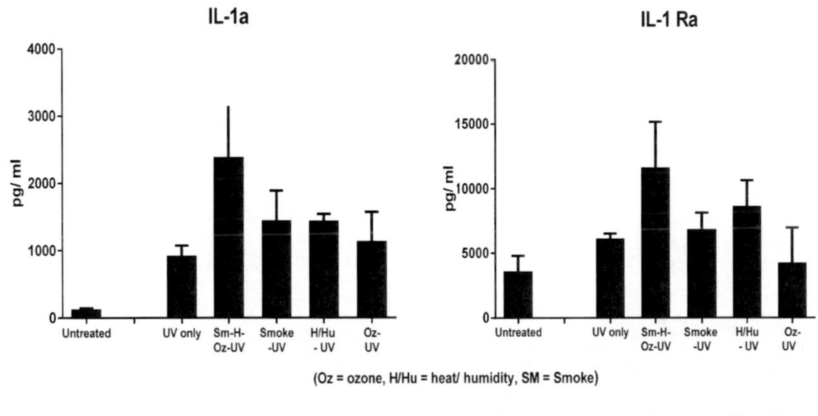

Figure 3b. Each individual stressor (ozone, heat humidity, smoke) when combined with UV displayed little to slight increase in the levels of pro-inflammatory cytokines. However, a combination of all the stressors with UV resulted in maximal induction of cytokines.

Ingredients to Protect Skin against Environmental Damage

Skin is exposed to many different types of environmental stressors including UV, pollution, heat, cold and wind. Multiple approaches are necessary to protect the skin against the damaging effects. A variety of ingredients used in topical products to address the environmental damage will be discussed.

Table 1. Categories of Ingredients to Protect against Environmental Aggressors

UV Filters		
UVB Filters	***UVB/short UVA Filters***	***UVA Filters***
Homosalate-UVB	Oxybenzone- UVB/short UVA	Avobenzone- UVA
Octisalate-UVB	Titanium Dioxide- UVB/sometimes short UVA	Zinc Oxide-UVB/UVA
Octocrylene-UVB		
Octinoxate- UVB		-
Antioxidants		
Vitamins	***Plants***	***Other***
Vitamin E	Ginseng	BHT
Vitamin C	Curcuma	
Vitamin A (and derivatives)	Ginkgo	
	Rosemary	
	Grape	
	Ginger	
	Garlic	
	Kiwi	
	Papaya	
	Blackberry	
	Green Tea	
	Beta carotene	

Skin Protectants/Conditioning		
Humectants	***Occlusive Agents***	***Emollients***
Glycerin	Petrolatum	Shea Butter
Urea	Lanolin	Dimethicone
Sodium PCA	Mineral oil	Linoleic Acid
Sorbitol	Castor oil	Stearic Acid
Panthenol	Safflower oil	Stearyl Alcohol
Propylene Glycol		Behenyl Alcohol
Butylene Glycol		Cetyl Alcohol
	Chelating Agents	
	Disodium EDTA	
	Tetrasodium EDTA	
	Alteromonas Ferment Filtrate	
	Anti-Inflammatory	
	Dipotassium Glycyrrhizate	
	Bisabolol	
	Allantoin	
	Ilex Paraguariensis Leaf Extract	
	Chrysanthemum Parthenium (Feverfew) Flower/Leaf/Stem Juice	
	Chamomilla Recutita (Matricaria) Extract	

Anti-Inflammatory		
	Zingiber Officinale (Ginger) Root Extract	
	Sodium Cocoyl Amino Acids; Sarcosine; Potassium Aspartate; Magnesium Aspartate	
	Portulaca Oleracea Extract	
	Other	
	Charcoal	
	Moringa Pterygosperma Seed Extract	
	Nylon-12	
	Polymethyl Methacrylate	
	Silica	

UV Filters

Topical Sunscreens can reduce the UV-induced formation of free radicals in skin and protect skin from oxidative damage. Singlet oxygen can be generated from the action of UVA (320 – 400 nm) and endogenous photosensitizers, such as porphyrins and flavins [28], which can produce DNA damage [29]. Irradiation with minimally erythemic doses of UVB (290 - 320 nm) also generates increases in Thymine-Thymine DNA damage [30]. Organic sunscreen filters absorb UV radiation which limits production of reactive oxidative species (ROS) and DNA damage. UVB filters contribute only marginally to the reduction of ROS. UVA filters are more effective in reducing free radical injury to the skin than UVB filters [31]. Therefore, in order to protect the skin against injury caused directly from UVB Thymine-Thymine DNA damage and UVA free radical generation in the dermis, it is necessary to use photostable broad spectrum UVA/UVB filters as the first line of defense.

The most common UVB absorbing sunscreens used in the US are Homosalate, Octisalate, Octocrylene, Octinoxate, Ensulizole, Oxybenzone, Titanium Dioxide and Zinc Oxide. In the US there are limitations to UVA approved sunscreens. Oxybenzone and some grades of Titanium Dioxide give short range UVA protection, while only Zinc Oxide and Avobenzone give full range UVA absorption. Some combinations of sunscreens are not FDA monograph approved, yielding an even smaller pallet of ingredients. In order to absorb the full UVA range, a formula must contain either Avobenzone or Zinc Oxide. Avobenzone loses absorption efficacy as a result of photoisomerization from the enol to the keto form and /or photodegradation. In order to maintain UVA photoprotection, a photostabilizer such as Octocrylene must be added to Avobenzone. Recently photostable broad spectrum UVA studies have been reported and technologies such as Helioplex® have been marketed [32].

Antioxidants

Antioxidants play an important role in protecting the skin from oxidative stress from UV, pollution, cold, and heat. Ozone is a strong oxidizing agent which has been shown to deplete the antioxidant levels within the outermost skin layer, the stratum corneum, as well as induce the oxidation of lipids and proteins. Cigarette smoke not only contains peroxy radicals but also contains nitric oxide which can facilitate conversion of peroxy radicals into the more highly reactive alkoxy and hydroxy radicals. Antioxidants are molecules that can neutralize free radicals by accepting or donating electron(s) to eliminate the unpaired radical. The antioxidant reacts directly with the reactive radical to destroy it, and either becomes a new free radical which is less active, longer-lived and less dangerous than the radical it has neutralized or other mechanisms terminate its radical status. Many have aromatic ring structures and are able to delocalize the unpaired electron. Another important function of antioxidants is to regulate ROS-related enzymes. Antioxidants may decrease the cellular level of free radicals either by inhibiting the activities or expressions of free radical generating enzymes such as NAD(P)H oxidase (NOX) and xanthine oxidase (XO) or by enhancing the activities and expressions of antioxidant enzymes such as superoxide dismutase (SOD), catalase (CAT) and glutathione peroxidase (GPX) [33].

Many vitamins are antioxidants and both Vitamin E (α-tocopherol) and Vitamin C are widely used in topical formulations. Naturally occurring vitamin E consists of eight distinct species, α-, β-, γ-, and δ- tocopherols, which differ in the number and location of methyl groups in their chroman ring, together with the corresponding unsaturated tocotrienols in which the phytyl side chain contains three olefinic double bonds [34]. The phytyl side chain of the tocopherols has three chiral centers so that synthetic α-tocopherol, sold as vitamin E supplements for instance, contains equal amounts of eight stereoisomers. Topically applied Vitamin E acetate (α-tocopherol acetate) has been shown to reduce the UVB-induced erythema and epidermal hyperplasia [35] and increase superoxide dismutase levels and the subsequent reduction in lipid peroxides [36]. In addition α-, γ-, and δ-tocopherols have been shown to significantly reduce thymine dimer formation [37]. Vitamin C (Ascorbic Acid) has a great redox potential and reacts with many reactive oxygen species and nitrogen species. Vitamin C can quench numerous forms of oxygen radicals such as singlet oxygen, superoxide, hydroxyl and water-soluble peroxyl radicals. In addition, Vitamin C can recycle the vitamin E radical (tocopheroxyl), thereby forming the ascorbyl radical and regenerating the active Vitamin E.

Many natural antioxidants come from fruit, vegetables, spices, grains and herbs such as green tea, grape, ginko, kiwi, rosemary and blackberries, however only a few are published in topical applications. They contain a variety of antioxidant compounds including but not limited to vitamins, carotenoid terpenoids and natural phenols. A newer approach of using antioxidants for skincare benefits involves boosting the skin's endogenous antioxidant machinery via activation of the Nrf2 pathway by natural actives like Feverfew [38]. An extract of Feverfew has also been shown to protect the skin from UV and environmental stressors [39].

Skin Protectants

The primary approach to protection from heat, cold and wind induced skin damage is to include a combination of humectants, emollients and occlusive agents to moisturize the skin and prevent skin barrier function disruption. Improving and strengthening the barrier function of the skin will decrease the water loss and improve the skin's moisture content which results in less cracking, rough and dry skin.

Humectants attract and bind water in the stratum corneum from either the dermis below or from the atmosphere. The molecules contain hydroxyl groups which allow them to hydrogen bond and attract water. Examples of humectants used in topical formulations are glycerin, propylene glycol, butylene glycol and sorbitol. Humectants have different water binding capacities and are chosen based on cost and the after feel imparted. Glycerin can be tacky and will need to be overcome in the formulation. Cosmetic suppliers have created humectant blends and modified ethoxylated methyl glucose ethers which give non-tacky aesthetics, however are more costly. The humectant blends include ingredients such as Sodium PCA, Sodium Lactate, Urea and polyquats.

Occlusive agents increase the skin's moisture content by providing a hydrophobic barrier over the skin to decrease epidermal water loss. Occlusives can diffuse into the intracellular lipid domains, increasing their efficacy. Petrolatum is the most effective occlusive agent, followed by lanolin, mineral oil and other oils and waxes. Most occlusive agents leave a greasy, heavy residue on the skin and therefore are sometimes not preferred.

Emollients are a large class of ingredients which can soften and condition the skin. They contain a wide range of chemicals from liquid silicones, esters and oils to solid esters, fatty alcohols, fatty acids and butters. Emollients can be grouped by their spreadability which allows for varying ranges of aesthetics. Essential fatty acids and fatty alcohols similar to those found in the skin, like lineolic acid and stearic acid, can improve skin's barrier function. Shea butter is used to improve and strengthen the skin's barrier. Shea butter is extracted from *Vitellaria paradoxa*, also known as the Shea Tree, which grows in Africa. The greenish shea butter is extracted from its nuts, which are similar to avocados. Shea butter has moisturizing and skin-protection properties. It contains a number of phenols including gallic acid, catechin, epicatechin, epicatechin gallate, gallocatechin and epigallocatechin gallate as well as quercetin and trans-cinnamic acid [40]. Shea butter is most often used for its emollient properties as an adjunctive for the care of itchy dry or compromised skin [41].

The combination of humectants, occlusive agents and emollients provides complementary activity to prevent skin barrier function disruption which can reduce the loss of hydration caused by heat, cold and wind.

Chelating Agents

As previously discussed, heavy metals like iron, copper, cadmium and arsenic are common air pollutants. These metals can catalyze the general formation of free-radicals via the Fenton reaction. Many antioxidants can act as pro-oxidants in metal-catalyzed oxidation therefore controlling metal ion contamination is recommended. It is important to chelate heavy metals such as cadmium and lead thus limiting the damages caused by toxic chemicals.

In topical formulations chelating agents such as EDTA's primary role is to protect the formulation by sequestering and decreasing the reactivity of metal ions that may be present in a product. Limited research has been done to determine their role in chelating heavy metals from pollution on the skin, however if investigated they may provide a benefit.

Anti-Inflammatory

UV irradiation, pollution, heat, cold and wind induce the expression of pro-inflammatory cytokines which triggers inflammation and can result in erythema. Many topical cosmetic ingredients can block pro-inflammatory cytokines which can be used to both prevent and treat erythema. Topical anti-inflammatory ingredients can reduce redness and soothe the skin.

Bisabolol is an example of a topical anti-inflammatory agent commonly added to sunscreen products and it is effective at preventing UV light erythema in addition to speeding up the erythema disappearance. Feverfew PFE can reduce the release of pro-inflammatory mediators through inhibitions of enzymes involved in production and regulation of inflammation, and also protect skin cells against UV-induced DNA damage [42]. Portulaca extract reduces skin erythema, relieves irritation and soothes skin through NO Synthesis Inhibition and 5-lipoxygenase Inhibition. Brazilian Green tea, Yerba Mate (Ilex Paraguariensis) is used as a topical anti-inflammatory in suncare products. Yerba Mate as compared to other teas has a higher concentration of saponins which can be attributed to the anti-inflammatory properties [43]. Dipotassium Glycyrrhizate is a compound extracted from liquorice root and contains saponins, flavonoids, chalcones, isoflavones, coumarins, stilbenoids for anti-inflammatory applications. It is a water soluble compound and can therefore be added to products where clarity or solubility is a concern.

Other

In addition to the categories mentioned above, there are other ingredients that can help protect against the five aggressors. By creating a physical barrier on the skin, pollution can be filtered out so it does not reach the skin. Examples of filters could be charcoal and Moringa Oleifera. Recent research has shown that topical application of Moringa oleifera was shown to protect the skin surface from coal particle pollution as evidenced with video microscopy. A biopsy test shows a marked reduction of HSP27 (a stress marker) levels in skin concurrently challenged with cigarette smoke and treated with 3% Moringa oleifera (studies conducted by BASF - Laboratoires Sérobiologiques, Division De Cognis France). Moringa seeds are rich in fatty acids such as Arachidic, Oleic, Palmitic, Stearic and Behenic acids, but also active substances such as Quercetin (a well-known metal chelator and cell protector), Tocopherol (a known anti-inflammation/anti-oxidation compound), and Ascorbic acid. Moringa Oleifera seeds are used to remove environmental pollutants from water. Moringa is used to filter water in some countries.

A physical barrier created by solid powders such as Polymethyl Methacrylate, Nylon-12 or Silica can prevent airborne particles from attaching to the surface of the skin. Limited research has been done in this area.

When protecting the skin against the five aggressors of UV light, pollution, heat, cold and wind it is important to combine technologies of different modes of action. The different pathways can protect the skin from direct and indirect damage as well as repair the skin. A multipronged approach will yield the most effective topical formulations. It is important to strengthen the skin's barrier and actively defend against pollutants and UV light.

Clinical Studies on Skin Damage from 5 Environmental Aggressors -Pollution, Natural Sunlight, Heat, Cold and Wind

The cumulative effect of 5 environmental aggressors (pollution, natural sunlight, heat, cold and wind) on skin was recently investigated in a randomized clinical study of 26 subjects ages 18 or older, Fitzpatrick types II-III [44]. 13 subjects used a lotion containing a combination of antipollution/anti-oxidant ingredients along with SPF25, and the remaining 13 subjects were assigned a lotion-only control formulation for 8 weeks. The environmental aggressors are generated using the following methods: Pollution (ozone, sulfur dioxide, PAH) was generated by exposing subjects to burning charcoal and wood in an open grill outdoors for a 20 minute period. Ultraviolet light (UVR) was generated by exposure to natural sunlight for a 20 minute period. Cold was generated by exposure to ice packs for two cycles of 10 minutes. Wind was generated by exposure to fans for a 20 minute period. Heat was generated by outdoor sun exposure for a 20 minute period. Clinical grading was assessed to evaluate photo-aging skin parameters (Figure 4). Biopsies were also taken from the lower back of 6 subjects that additionally applied test material to the lower back using an open application technique for 4 days prior to biopsy collection. Three punch biopsies (3mm) were obtained per subject, one treated site exposed to environmental aggressors, one untreated site exposed to environmental aggressors and one untreated, unexposed naïve site. All biopsies are analyzed for the following biomarkers: thymine dimers, MMP-1, sunburn cell counts, IL-1α and IL-8.

Biopsy Study analysis suggest that cell death and DNA damage levels in treated skin is close to the levels in naïve (not aggressed, not treated) skin, and much lower than the levels in skin that has been subjected to the aggressors without protection. After only 4 days of treatment with lotion formulation containing a combination of antipollution/anti-oxidant/SPF25 ingredients, the skin was significantly protected at a biological level from cumulative assault by 5 environmental aggressors. Taken together, these results collectively demonstrate that environmental aggressors can induce skin damage that can contribute to accelerated skin aging. A topical formulation containing a combination of antipollution/anti-oxidant/SPF25 ingredients, significantly improved signs of pollution-induced aging, and protected the skin against damage produced by the combination of solar UV radiation and environmental stressors.

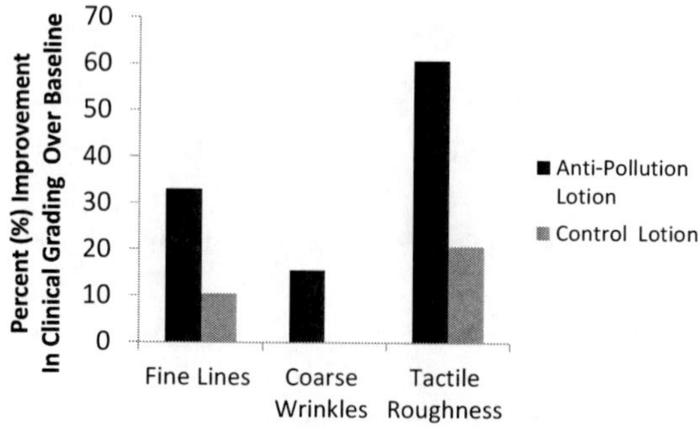

Figure 4. In an 8-week , placebo-controlled study, subjects who used a lotion formulation containing a combination of antipollution/anti-oxidant/SPF25 ingredients on their faces saw significant improvements in fine lines, coarse wrinkles, tactile roughness, as compared to the placebo.

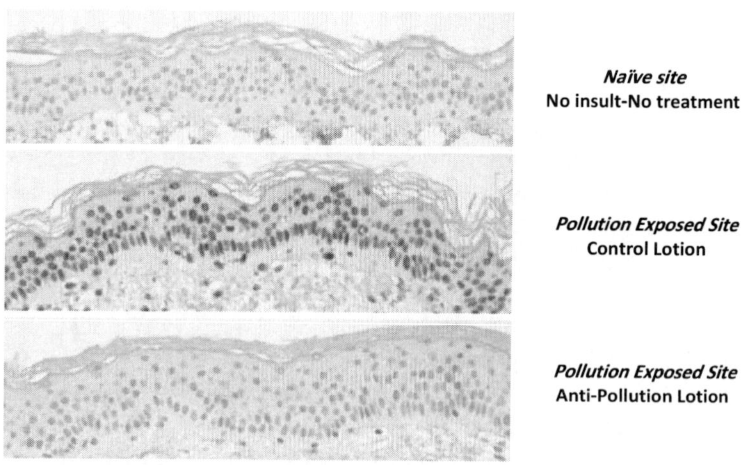

Figure 5a. Thymine dimers staining show comparable levels at naïve site (no pollution) and the site exposed to pollution and treated with the lotion formulation containing a combination of antipollution/anti-oxidant/SPF25 ingredients. In contrast the pollution exposed site treated with control lotion formulation showed very high levels of DNA damage. This indicates a strong protective effect by the test product, treatment with antipollution formulation protected the epidermis from the cumulative effects of environmental aggression.

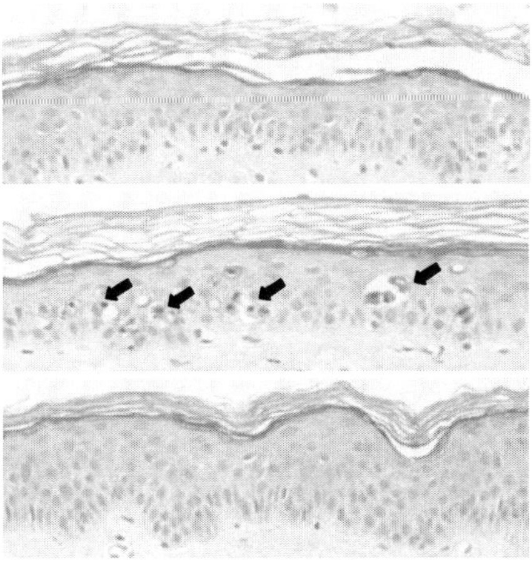

Figure 5b. Staining for apoptotic cells show comparable levels at naïve site (no pollution) and the site exposed to pollution and treated with the lotion formulation containing a combination of antipollution/anti-oxidant/SPF25 ingredients. In contrast the pollution exposed site treated with control emollient formulation showed very high levels of cell death (apoptosis).

Conclusion

Skin is the primary interface between the body and surrounding atmosphere, and is therefore our first line of defense from environmental pollutants and other aggressors. Increasing evidence shows that people are exposed to greater levels of pollution and environmental aggression. Acute exposure to pollution can induce oxidative damage and inflammation in skin cells, while chronic exposure to pollution has been shown to exacerbate signs of skin damage and aging, including fine lines, wrinkles, formation of pigmented spots [17], and also damage to the skin barrier [45, 46]. Furthermore, as shown in figure 6 below, exposure to everyday pollution can synergistically damage skin, especially enhancing the UV induced skin damage, with pollution doubling the skin damage from UV alone. Topical formulations may provide some protection and remediation for skin exposed to everyday pollution. Holistic skin protection from everyday pollution can be achieved utilizing a combination of sun filters, anti-oxidant/anti-inflammatories, and physical blockers to mitigate the skin damage when exposed to the 5 environmental aggressors (pollution, natural sunlight, heat, cold and wind). Taken together, the cumulative effect of exposing skin to everyday pollution can affect skin physiology, alter the skin barrier and may accelerate the skin aging process.

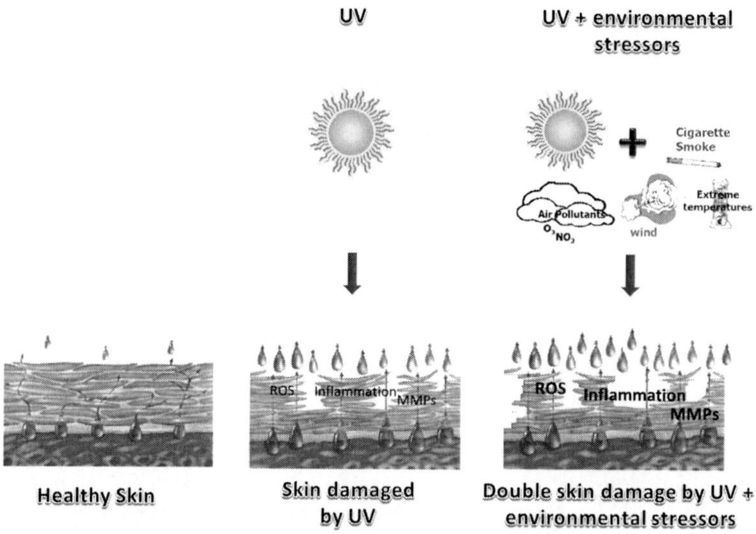

Figure 6. Proposed model showing that the cumulative effects of environmental stressors along with UV double the damage to skin by inducing higher levels of ROS, inflammation, and MMPs.

References

[1] Drakaki, E., Dessinioti, C. & Antoniou, C. V. (2014) Air Pollution and the skin. *Frontiers in Environmental Science*, *2*.

[2] Uitto, J (2008) The role of elastin and collagen in cutaneous aging: intrinsic aging versus photoexposure. *J Drugs Dermatol*, *7*, s12-16.

[3] Christensen, K., Iachina, M., Rexbye, H., Tomassini, C., Frederiksen, H., et al. (2004) "Looking old for your age": genetics and mortality. *Epidemiology*, *15*, 251-252.

[4] Guyuron, B., Rowe, D. J., Weinfeld A. B., Eshraghi Y., Fathi A., et al. (2009) Factors contributing to the facial aging of identical twins. *Plast Reconstr Surg.*, *123*, 1321-1331.

[5] Fisher, G. J., Kang, S., Varani, J., Bata-Csorgo, Z., Wan, Y., et al. (2002) Mechanisms of photoaging and chronological skin aging. *Arch Dermatol*, *138*, 1462-1470.

[6] Jenkins, G (2002) Molecular mechanisms of skin ageing. *Mech Ageing Dev*, *123*, 801-810.

[7] Fligiel, S. E., Varani, J., Datta, S. C., Kang, S., Fisher, G. J., et al. (2003) Collagen degradation in aged/photodamaged skin in vivo and after exposure to matrix metalloproteinase-1 in vitro. *J Invest Dermatol*, *120*, 842-848.

[8] Kligman, L. H., Akin, F. J. & Kligman, A. M (1985) The contributions of UVA and UVB to connective tissue damage in hairless mice. *J Invest Dermatol*, *84*, 272-276.

[9] Chung, J. H., Seo, J. Y., Lee, M. K., Eun, H. C., Lee, J. H., et al. (2002) Ultraviolet modulation of human macrophage metalloelastase in human skin in vivo. *J Invest Dermatol*, *119*, 507-512.

[10] Fisher, G. J., Datta, S. C., Talwar, H. S., Wang, Z. Q., Varani, J., et al. (1996) Molecular basis of sun-induced premature skin ageing and retinoid antagonism. *Nature*, *379*, 335-339.

[11] Fisher GJ., Wang ZQ., Datta SC., Varani J., Kang S., et al. (1997) Pathophysiology of premature skin aging induced by ultraviolet light. *N Engl J Med*, *337*, 1419-1428.

[12] Li N., Sioutas C., Cho A., Schmitz D., Misra C., et al. (2003) Ultrafine particulate pollutants induce oxidative stress and mitochondrial damage. *Environ Health Perspect*, *111*, 455-460.

[13] Lademann, J., Schaefer, H., Otberg, N., Teichmann, A., Blume-Peytavi U., et al. (2004) [Penetration of microparticles into human skin]. Hautarzt 55: 1117-1119.

[14] Burke, K. E. & Wei, H. (2009) Synergistic damage by UVA radiation and pollutants. Toxicol Ind Health, *25*, 219-224.

[15] Donaldson, K., Tran, L., Jimenez, L. A., Duffin, R., Newby, D. E., et al. (2005) Combustion-derived nanoparticles: a review of their toxicology following inhalation exposure. *Part Fibre Toxicol*, *2*, 10.

[16] Wan, R., Mo, Y., Zhang, X., Chien, S., Tollerud, D. J., et al. (2008) Matrix metalloproteinase-2 and -9 are induced differently by metal nanoparticles in human monocytes: The role of oxidative stress and protein tyrosine kinase activation. *Toxicol Appl Pharmacol*, *233*, 276-285.

[17] Vierkotter, A., Schikowski, T., Ranft, U., Sugiri, D., Matsui, M., et al. Airborne particle exposure and extrinsic skin aging. *J Invest Dermatol*, *130*, 2719-2726.

[18] Solly, S. (1856) Clinical Lectures ON PARALYSIS. *The Lancet*, *68*, 641-643.

[19] Gilchrest, B. & Krutmann, J (2006) Premature Skin Aging by Infrared Radiation, Tobacco Smoke and Ozone. Skin Aging: *Springer Berlin Heidelberg*. 45-53.

[20] Lahmann, C., Bergemann, J., Harrison, G. & Young, AR (2001) Matrix metalloproteinase-1 and skin ageing in smokers. *Lancet*, *357*, 935-936.

[21] Yin, L., Morita, A., Tsuji, T. (2000) Alterations of extracellular matrix induced by tobacco smoke extract. *Arch Dermatol Res*., 292, 188-194.

[22] Doshi, D. N., Hanneman, K. K., Cooper, K. D (2007) Smoking and skin aging in identical twins. *Arch Dermatol*, *143*, 1543-1546.

[23] Rasmussen, C., Gratz, K., Liebel, F., Southall, M., Garay, M., et al. The StrataTest(R) human skin model, a consistent in vitro alternative for toxicological testing. *Toxicol In Vitro*, *24*, 2021-2029.

[24] Valacchi, G., Pagnin, E., Okamoto, T., Corbacho, A. M., Olano, E., et al. (2003) Induction of stress proteins and MMP-9 by 0.8 ppm of ozone in murine skin. *Biochem Biophys Res Commun*, *305*, 741-746.

[25] McCarthy JT., Pelle E., Dong K., Brahmbhatt K., Yarosh D., et al. Effects of ozone in normal human epidermal keratinocytes. *Exp Dermatol*, *22*, 360-361.

[26] Afaq, F., Zaid, M. A., Pelle, E., Khan, N., Syed, D. N., et al. (2009) Aryl hydrocarbon receptor is an ozone sensor in human skin. *J Invest Dermatol*, *129*, 2396-2403.

[27] Roure, R., Lanctin, M., Nollent, V., Bertin, C Methods to Assess the Protective Efficacy of Emollients against Climatic and Chemical Aggressors. *Dermatol Res Pract*, 2012, 864734.

[28] Cadet, J., Berger, M., Douki, T., Morin, B., Raoul, S., et al. (1997) Effects of UV and visible radiation on DNA-final base damage. *Biol Chem*, *378*, 1275-1286.

[29] Ravanat, J. L., Di Mascio, P., Martinez, G. R., Medeiros, M. H., Cadet, J. (2000) Singlet oxygen induces oxidation of cellular DNA. *J Biol Chem*, *275*, 40601-40604.

[30] Pelle, E., Huang, X., Mammone, T., Marenus, K., Maes, D., et al. (2003) Ultraviolet-B-induced oxidative DNA base damage in primary normal human epidermal keratinocytes and inhibition by a hydroxyl radical scavenger. *J Invest Dermatol*, *121*, 177-183.

[31] Herrling, T., Jung, K., Chatelain, E., Langenauer, M Radical Skin/Sun Protection Factor RSFâ€“.

[32] Cole, C., Appa, Y. & Ou-Yang, H. (2014) A broad spectrum high-SPF photostable sunscreen with a high UVA-PF can protect against cellular damage at high UV exposure doses. *Photodermatol Photoimmunol Photomed*, 30, 212-219.

[33] Lu, J. M., Lin, P. H., Yao, Q., Chen, C. (2010) Chemical and molecular mechanisms of antioxidants: experimental approaches and model systems. *J Cell Mol Med*, 14, 840-860.

[34] Kayden, H. J. & Traber, M. G (1993) Absorption, lipoprotein transport, and regulation of plasma concentrations of vitamin E in humans. *J Lipid Res*, *34*, 343-358.

[35] Trevithick, J. R., Xiong, H., Lee, S., Shum, D. T., Sanford, S. E., et al. (1992) Topical tocopherol acetate reduces post-UVB, sunburn-associated erythema, edema, and skin sensitivity in hairless mice. *Arch Biochem Biophys*, 296, 575-582.

[36] Lopez-Torres, M., Thiele, J. J., Shindo, Y., Han, D. & Packer, L. (1998) Topical application of alpha-tocopherol modulates the antioxidant network and diminishes ultraviolet-induced oxidative damage in murine skin. *Br J Dermatol*, *138*, 207-215.

[37] McVean, M. & Liebler, D. C (1999) Prevention of DNA photodamage by vitamin E compounds and sunscreens: roles of ultraviolet absorbance and cellular uptake. *Mol Carcinog.*, *24*, 169-176.

[38] Rodriguez, K. J., Wong, H. K., Oddos, T., Southall, M., Frei, B., et al. A purified feverfew extract protects from oxidative damage by inducing DNA repair in skin cells via a PI3-kinase-dependent Nrf2/ARE pathway. *J Dermatol Sci*, *72*, 304-310.

[39] Martin, K., Sur, R., Liebel, F., Tierney, N., Lyte, P., et al. (2008). Parthenolide-depleted Feverfew (Tanacetum parthenium) protects skin from UV irradiation and external aggression. *Arch Dermatol Res*, *300*, 69-80.

[40] Maranz, S., Wiesman, Z. & Garti, N (2003) Phenolic constituents of shea (Vitellaria paradoxa) kernels. *J Agric Food Chem*, *51*, 6268-6273.

[41] Belibi, S. E. S. D. & Olson, N., (2009) The Use of Shea Butter as an Emollient for Eczema. *Journal of Allergy and Clinical Immunology*, *123*, S41.

[42] Southall, M. D., Kaur, S. & Mahmood, K. (2011) The botanical extract Feverfew PFE reduces DNA damage and induces DNA repair processes; Chen C, editor: Intech.

[43] Heck, C. I., de Mejia, E. G. (2007) Yerba Mate Tea (Ilex paraguariensis): a comprehensive review on chemistry, health implications, and technological considerations. *J Food Sci.*, *72*, R138-151.

[44] Garay, M. P., Dari, Kaur., Simarna, Bhattacharyya., Surjya, Barkovic, Sylvia, (2011) Ability of a topical formulation containing botanical antioxidants to mitigate synergistic skin damaging effects of ultraviolet radiation and environmental aggressors and improve skin barrier. Poster Abstracts American Academy of Dermatology 72nd *Annual Meeting*, *64*, AB23.

[45] Krutmann, J., Liu, W., Li, L., Pan, X., Crawford, M., et al. Pollution and skin: from epidemiological and mechanistic studies to clinical implications. *J Dermatol Sci.*, *76*, 163-168.

[46] Vierkotter, A., Krutmann, *J Environmental influences on skin aging and ethnic-specific manifestations. Dermatoendocrinol*, *4*, 227-231.

In: Skin Aging and Photoaging
Editor: Emanuel Graham
ISBN: 978-1-63482-907-6

Chapter 4

New Insights on the Role of Inflammation in Regulation of Skin Aging

Ali Fassih, Anne-Sophie Brillouet, Dianne Rossetti, Simarna Kaur and Michael D. Southall[*]
Johnson and Johnson Consumer Companies, Inc.,
Skillman, NJ, US

Abstract

Our skin is under continuous assault from a variety of damaging environmental factors including ultraviolet irradiation and atmospheric pollutants. The skin aging process is governed by changes in the epidermal, dermal-epidermal junction and dermal compartments. Extracellular matrix (ECM) proteins, which are the major component of dermis, constitute an important target for intrinsic and extrinsic aging related alterations. Extrinsic factors, particularly sunlight, have been demonstrated to accelerate the aging process, resulting in elastosis, inflammation, and increased matrix protein degradation which cumulatively manifest as photo-damage and accelerated skin aging. The pro-inflammatory NF-κB (nuclear factor kappa-light-chain-enhancer of

[*] Corresponding author: Michael Southall, Johnson & Johnson Consumer Companies, Inc. Phone: 908-874-2318 ; Fax: 908-874-1209, Email: msoutha@its.jnj.com.

activated B cells) pathway is one of the key signaling pathways that have been implicated in the regulation of skin ECM production. The NF-kB pathway can be activated by sunlight and reactive oxygen species, and has been reported to be the final common pathway for the conversion of environmental insults into inflammation in the skin. Recently studies report that the activity of NF-κB in the skin increases as a function of age, suggesting that sub-clinical levels of inflammation in our skin increase as we age. The direct link between NF-κB activation and suppression of matrix proteins such as elastin and collagen in dermal fibroblasts has been demonstrated, suggesting that NF-κB may be a causative factor in extrinsic aging by contributing to an acceleration of the skin aging process. Furthermore, when NF-κB is active in dermal fibroblasts, the ECM inducing activity of anti-aging actives such as Retinol (Vitamin A) are significantly reduced. A double-blind clinical anti-aging study reported that an inhibitor of NF-κB resulted in significant clinical improvement in facial wrinkles and other parameters associated with skin aging and pigmentation. In addition, an NF-κB inhibitor was shown to increase the effectiveness of Retinol, increasing Retinol bioactivity and resulting in an increased clinical anti-aging efficacy. By inhibiting a major pathway responsible for the inflammatory response in skin and the subsequent loss of matrix proteins, inhibition of NF-κB has been shown to improve the signs of aging in photo-damaged skin. Taken together, NF-κB inhibitors appear to have great potential as a dermatological tool that can mitigate the signs of premature aging in patients.

Introduction

Skin and Aging Process

Skin is the largest and one of the most complex organs in human body, accounting for almost 15% of total body weight. It serves as an important environmental interface and thus acts as a first line of defense against various environmental insults. Skin is organized into three main layers, epidermis, dermis and subcutaneous layer. The epidermis, an outermost avascular layer, is formed by keratinocytes at the epidermal basal layer that differentiate into corneocytes at the outer layer of the epidermis. The dermis lies below the epidermis separated by a basement membrane and is composed mainly of fibroblasts. The primary function of skin is to constitute an efficient barrier to protect the organism both from water evaporation and from damage, as such skin is exposed to many external and internal aggressors.

Intrinsically aged skin exhibits signs of damage such as reduced elastin content and a general decline in a variety of cell populations [1]. Because of skin aging, skin becomes increasing thin, dry, pale, and wrinkled over time [2, 3]. Factors in both the epidermis and the dermis contribute to the thinning of older skin, with a reduction in keratinocytes observed in the epidermis and decease in the amount and organisation of the extracellular matrix (ECM) in the dermis [2, 3]. The ECM of the dermis is composed primarily of collagen, elastin, proteoglycans and glycosaminoglycans with dermal fibroblasts embedded within. It is the degeneration of collagen and elastin over time and the resulting loss of strength and elasticity that causes intrinsic skin aging. This intrinsic skin aging process is inherent with the passage of time; however, it is exacerbated by the presence of many extrinsic factors which can induce skin aging.

Skin under External Aggression and Inflammation

Our skin is first barrier between our bodies and the environment, providing protection from the environment's chemical and physical challenges. Geographic location and lifestyle factors such as ultraviolet radiation, extreme hot and cold temperatures, dryness, and air pollution impose constant challenges to the skin barrier, and can contribute to skin aging. To function effectively the skin must be resilient in overcoming the detrimental effects of these assaults. Generally, environmental stressors result in formation of oxidative compounds, eventually leading to oxidative stress, inflammation, and cellular damage, all of which ultimately contribute to degradation of skin matrix proteins which manifests as signs of skin aging, such as wrinkles.

Intrinsic aging, linked to genetic factors, is an inevitable fate for all skin. However, it is widely accepted that extrinsic, external aggression-induced aging accounts for the majority of the visible signs of skin aging. Indeed, between 40%-90% of the aged appearance of the skin is attributed to extrinsic aging [4, 5]. To isolate the effects of extrinsic skin aging, Guyuron et al. studied the effect of UV exposure and cigarette smoke on the apparent age of identical twins [6]. The researchers showed that higher apparent age correlated with increased outdoor activity and cigarette smoke. They also demonstrated an increased aged appearance for participants who used less sunscreen.

Several lines of evidence suggest that extrinsic aging is mediated by inflammation. Inflammation is the natural protective mechanism to correcting physiological challenges such as infection, DNA damage, and wound repair. However, due to the destructive nature of inflammation, protection comes at the cost of tissue damage. An initial step in translating environmental signals to inflammation is through the formation of highly reactive oxidative compounds. Though extremely short-lived, these reactive oxygen species (ROS) can confer direct damage to tissues. Furthermore, these compounds may be quasi-stabilized by formation of secondary oxidative molecules such as lipid peroxides, which may diffuse to surrounding tissues, resulting in deeper inflammatory tissue damage. To some extent, the skin is equipped with a biochemical system of antioxidant release pathways that offset oxidative damage. However, chronic exposure leads to accumulation of these oxidants and eventually overwhelms endogenous antioxidant supplies, leading to oxidative stress, and inflammation. Consequently, the onset of inflammation promotes additional generation of oxidative compounds as well as enzymes that degrade the skin matrix proteins (e.g., matrix metalloproteinases, MMP). As such, an inflammatory response arising from environmental exposure may lead to a vicious cycle that amplifies the effects of the environment on tissue damage and skin aging.

The most significant environmental challenges, with respect to skin aging, are from UV radiation, by way of sun exposure, and air pollution, including exposure to cigarette smoke. Chronic exposure to these factors has been shown to result in cumulative damage to skin constituents, leading to premature skin thinning, wrinkling, and hyperpigmentation which contribute to the aged appearance of the skin [7-9]. There are reduced levels of extracellular matrix proteins, such as collagen and elastin, in aged skin. Additionally, there is a diminished capacity to regenerate ECM proteins in aged skin, magnifying the effect of inflammation on skin aging for older individuals.

Below are reviewed the effects of various environmental stressors, all of which may lead to oxidative stress, inflammation, and MMP release, ultimately resulting in diminished extracellular matrix protein constituents, which is a primary cause of aged appearance of skin. This is the currently accepted central paradigm of extrinsic skin aging.

UV Exposure and Skin Inflammation

It is widely accepted that cumulative UV exposure is the major cause of premature skin aging in today's middle aged and elderly population, leading to so-called photoaging, ultimately by means of damage to the skin's connective tissue. The relatively recent depletion of the protective stratospheric ozone layer increases the susceptibility of the skin to UV damage. The subset of UV radiation involved in skin aging is broken into two classifications, each with varying biochemical effects. The higher energy UV-B (280-315 nm) affects the outermost layer of the skin, whereas the lower energy UV-A (315-400 nm) penetrates beyond the epidermis.

Kligman et al., demonstrated elastic fiber damage and dermal tissue hypertrophy following either UVA or UVB exposure [10]. They also demonstrated summation of the deleterious effects when co-administered. As solar radiation inseparably contains UVA and UVB, this work highlights the need for photoprotection against both bands to prevent damaging effects of UV (broad spectrum protection).

Ultraviolet radiation elicits tissue and cellular damage either directly via immediate interaction between photons and skin constituents, or indirectly, through generation of reactive oxygen species (ROS). Direct UV damage may occur via cyclobutane-pyrimidine dimerization (CPD), leading to mutations during DNA replication. Direct photoreaction also results in formation of the most common DNA lesion, 8-oxo-guanine, causing mismatched replication and mutation. Indirect effects of UV result from the oxidative action of UV induced ROS on various skin constituents, including DNA, proteins, and lipids.

Whether by direct or indirect mechanisms, UV exposure induces inflammatory responses in the skin, leading to the release of ECM-degrading MMPs. It has been shown that even very low doses of UV radiation up-regulate AP-1 and NF-kB (Nuclear Factor Kappa-light-chain-enhancer of activated B cells) DNA binding, leading to induction of the MMPs, collagenase, 92-kd gelatinase, and stromelysin-1. Additionally UV exposure has been shown to increase MMP-3, MMP-9, and MMP-12 [11, 12]. Fisher et al., showed that controlled UV exposure of non-exposed skin resulted in 58% greater degradation of type I collagen fibrils compared to non-irradiated control skin in vivo [13]. Prolonged activity of MMPs in the skin leads to abnormal rates of dermal degradation of collagen and elastin which lead to premature aging.

Environmental Pollution and Skin Inflammation

Rapid industrialization has led to increased levels of environmental air pollution, particularly in highly populated metropolitan cities. Consequently, populations living in highly industrialized areas have been linked to having a higher incidence of certain health conditions such as cancer, and pulmonary and cardiovascular diseases. Air pollution has also been implicated in accelerating skin aging due to the pro-oxidant and pro-inflammatory nature of air pollutants.

Particulate Matter

Particulate matter (PM) is one such air pollutant. Characterized as nanoparticulate matter suspended in the air, such as those originating from fossil fuel combustion, PM's are a growing concern with potential to affect millions worldwide. In addition to their own inherent toxicity, PM's act as carriers for other detrimental environmental agents such as polycyclic aromatic hydrocarbons (PAH) and metals [14]. Due to their small size PMs penetrate into the skin and co-deliver adsorbed toxic agents [15]. Particulate matter has been postulated to induce ROS in skin [16]. Li et al., suggested that these particles may enter the mitochondria and initiate ROS generation [14]. Studies have not yet directly connected skin exposure to particulate matter and MMP release. However, it has been shown that metal nanoparticles do upregulate MMP-2, and MMP-9 induction in monocytes, via ROS generation [17]. Vierkotter et al., investigated the clinical influence of PM levels on inflammation and aging in 400 Caucasian women, indicating a correlation between a composite aging score and local particulate matter levels [18].

Ozone

Ozone is the major oxidative component of photochemical smog. It is known to rapidly degrade antioxidants, induce ROS, and initiate inflammation in exposed tissues, including respiratory epithelia and skin. Mice exposed to ozone levels comparable to levels observed in polluted cities exhibited increased lipid peroxidation, and increased MMP-9 expression and activity, in exposed skin [19].

Tobacco Smoke

Given that smoking tobacco products is strongly associated with many diseases including lung cancer, emphysema, and cardiovascular disease, it comes as no surprise that smokers physically appear older than their true age. Cigarette smoke has been associated with premature skin aging since the mid-1800s [20]. Oxidative compounds in cigarette smoke generate ROS upon exposure to lung and skin tissues. Similar to UV exposure, cigarette smoke initiates a cascade of events leading to inflammation, MMP release, and premature aging.

Cigarette smoke induces significantly greater MMP-1 gene expression in skin of smokers compared to non-smokers, implying systemic inflammatory effects of smoking [21]. Yin et al., demonstrated increased MMP3 mRNA in human fibroblasts following exposure to the water soluble fraction of tobacco smoke [22]. In addition, they showed that collagen biosynthesis was reduced by 40%. On the other hand, tissue inhibitors of matrix metalloproteinases (TIMP) were unaffected by exposure. The work exemplifies that smoking creates an imbalance of ECM processes detrimental to dermal collagen levels. Furthermore, a case study of identical twin sisters with similar lifestyle factors showed dramatic differences in severity of skin aging for the smoking twin compared to a non-smoking sister demonstrating the clinical relevance of the effects of smoke exposure [23].

MMPs and Aging

The MMP-mediated model of ECM deficiency is the most widely accepted model of extrinsic skin aging [13]. MMP release is a common step between the exposure to multiple environmental stressors and skin aging. MMP induction has been demonstrated in skin following exposure to UV, air pollution, and cigarette smoke. Other physiological conditions causing oxidative stresses and inflammation, such as psychological stress, chronic hyperallergenicity, metabolic syndrome, and skin dryness, may theoretically contribute to MMP-mediated skin aging.

The common final step in the inflammatory pathway leading to MMP release involves upregulation of NF-κB, as a response to increased inflammatory mediators such as IL- α, TNF-α, and ROS. It has been shown that inhibiting NF-κB reduces MMP release and stimulates production of ECM proteins, leading to opportunities for antiaging intervention therapies. The next section will discuss the role of NF-κB in inflammation and aging.

NF-κB and Inflammation

NF-κB was first described in 1986 as a nuclear factor essential for immunoglobulin κ light chain transcription in B cells [24]. Since that initial discovery, NF-κB has been found to be a primary mediator involved in regulating immune responses, apoptosis and cellular growth, as well as being present in inflammatory diseases such as arthritis and asthma [25]. The NF-κB family of transcription factors shares a high-conserved sequence of amino acids within their *amino terminus,* which contains a nuclear localization sequence that is involved in the dimerization with sequence-specific DNA binding and with the inhibitory IκB proteins.

In unstimulated cells, NF-κB-family proteins exist as heterodimers or homodimers that are sequestered in the cytoplasm in an inactive form by virtue of their association with a member of the IκB family of inhibitory proteins , most notably IκBα, IκBβ, and IκBγ [26, 27]. About 200 extracellular signals can lead to activation through the dissociation of NF-κB from the IκB proteins. These activating signals include viral and bacterial products, oxidative stress, pro-inflammatory cytokines including IL-1 and TNF-α, and phorbol esters [28-30, 31, 32], which result in the activation of the IκB kinase (IKK). UV radiation from sunlight induces IL-1 and TNF-α and creates reactive oxygen species that then leads to NF-κB-mediated inflammation [33, 34]. The kinase activity of IκK phosphorylates two serine residues (Ser32 and Ser36) on IκB proteins, which results in the ubiquitination and degradation of IκB by the proteasome. The degradation of IκB reveals the nuclear localization sequence of NF-κB [26]. Free NF-κB can then translocate to the nucleus and bind to a NF-κB *consensus* sequence present within the promoter region of target genes, thereby upregulating the expression of hundreds of genes, including cytokines (IL-1, -2, -6, etc.), immunoreceptors (immunoglobin kappa light chain, MHC class I, etc.), cellular adhesion molecules (ICAM-1, VCAM-1, ELAM-1), and many others[31].

In addition to the role in inflammation, the NF-κB pathway is a key regulator leading to excessive expression and subsequent activity of MMPs such as collagenase and elastase (MMPs 1, 3 and 9). The NF-κB pathway also further induces IL-1 and TNF-α, thus up-regulating its own pathway [35]. This feed forward mechanism can result in an amplification of inflammation and skin aging damage. The NF-κB pathway is therefore a primary factor in one of the processes mediating extrinsic skin aging, regulating the expression for matrix degrading proteins. In contrast, the second process mediating intrinsic skin aging, the age dependent decline in the skin's ability to produce matrix proteins such as elastin and collagen, and the etiology of this inhibition and putative role of NF-κB in skin aging, have not been well understood.

NF-κB Levels in Skin during Aging

Recent research studies have investigated the direct effects of NF-κB activation on ECM proteins which could suggest a role of NF-κB in the intrinsic aging process. If NF-κB is involved in the intrinsic skin aging process, then it would be speculated that levels of NF-κB could be expected to increase during the aging process. Studies on the cell aging process have reported that the NF-κB binding activity was found to be increased as a function of age [36, 1]. In fibroblasts isolated from human skin, the activity of NF-κB in skin of aged subjects showed that NF-κB was considerably more active in skin of older subjects (>51 years) compared with that of their younger counterparts (<50 years) as is shown in Figure 1 [38]. These results are consistent with a recent and more in-depth study reported by Bigot et al. that electromobility shift assays with a NF-κB consensus probe demonstrated that the DNA–protein complexes involving the P65 and P50 NF-κB subunits were prevalent in isolated fibroblasts obtained from skin biopsies and that the age of the skin donors was proportionally correlated with the NF-κB binding activity [39].

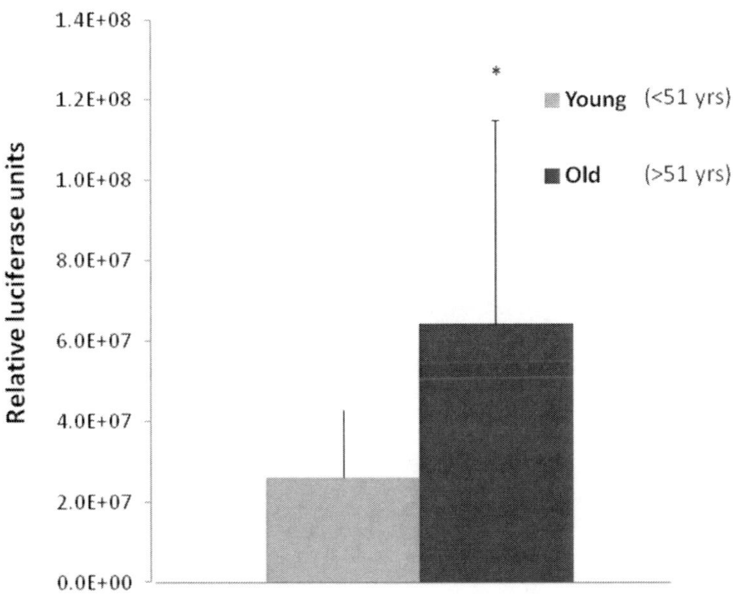

Figure 1. Aged fibroblasts display higher amounts and binding activity of NF-κB than young individuals. Human dermal fibroblasts derived from young (<50 years old; n=11) and older (>51 years old; n=10) donors were transiently transfected with pSV40-ß-gal, and the NF-κB Luciferase reporter construct. Values are mean ± SD expressed as relative luciferase units (RLU).

These results suggest that as we age, subclinical levels of inflammation in our skin are elevated, as evidenced by the increase in NF-κB levels with age, and support the hypothesis that NF-κB activation in skin may accelerate the skin-aging process.

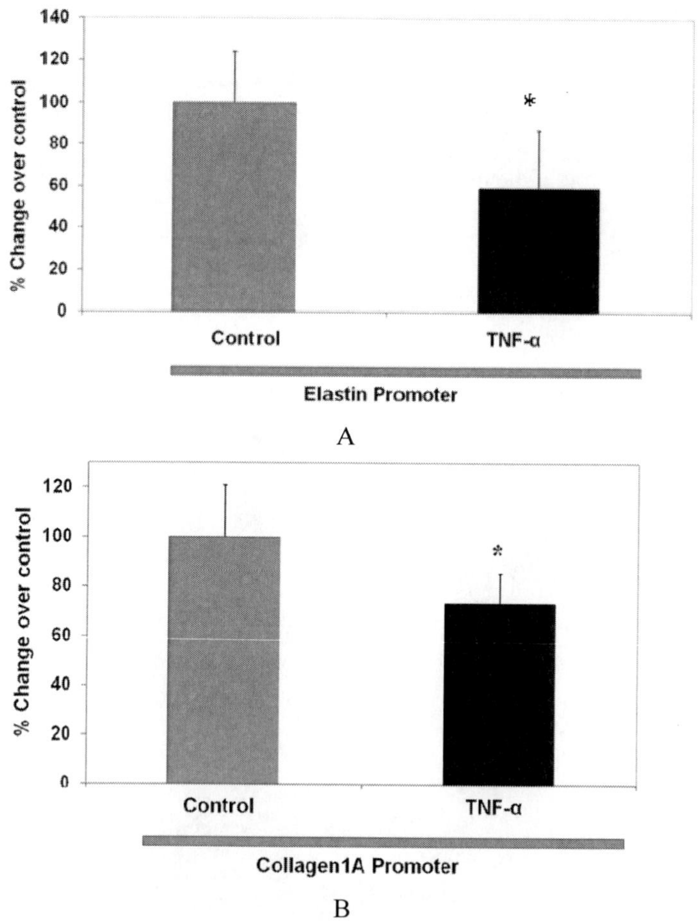

Figure 2. H9c2 cells transfected with the (a) Elastin or (b) Collagen1A promoters were treated with TNF-α for 24 hr to activate the NF-κB pathway, leading to suppression of Elastin and Collagen promoter levels. *$p<0.05$ compared to untreated control, using Student's t-test.

The induction of MMPs by activation of NF-κB pathway has been widely demonstrated; however, few studies have investigated the direct effects of NF-κB activation on ECM proteins. A direct connection was sought out by demonstrating the effects of NF-κB inhibition on ECM expression in vitro. Two inhibitors of NF-κB pathway: 4-hexyl-1, 3-phenylenediol (HP), which has been previously demonstrated to be a potent inhibitor of NF-κB activation [38, 40], and BAY-11-7082, a pharmacological inhibitor of NF-κB pathway, were shown to restore ECM levels in vitro (see Figures 2 -3).

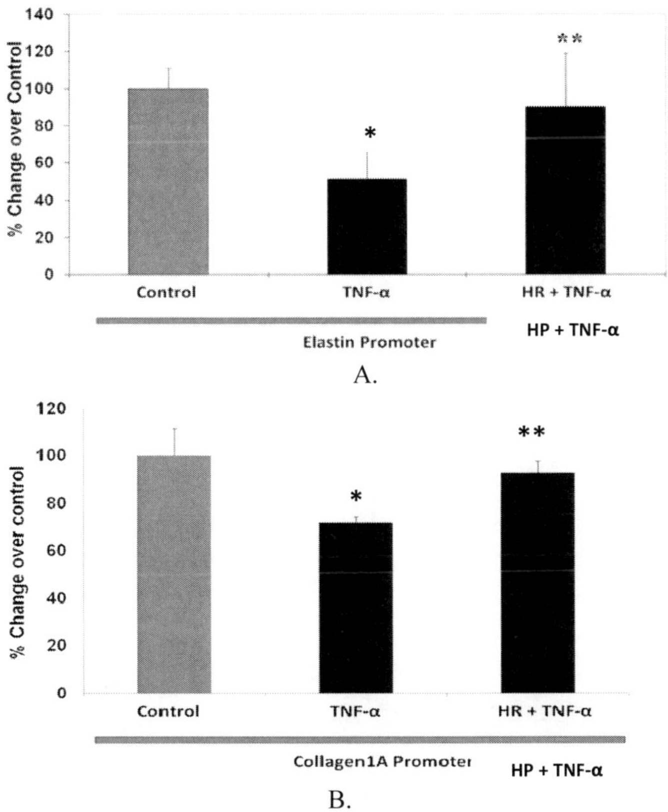

Figure 3. H9c2 cells were transfected with the Elastin (A) or Collagen1A (B) promoter followed by treatment with TNF-α in the absence or presence of HR for 24 hr. The downregulation of Collagen expression caused by activation of NF-κB was reversed in the presence of the inhibitor. *p<0.05 compared to untreated control. **p<0.05 compared to TNF-α treatment alone using Student's t-test.

NF-κB Inhibitors Boost the Bioactivity of Retinol by Blocking Inflammation

Retinol, a form of Vitamin A, has long been used as an anti-aging ingredient to reduce the signs of aging. Retinol improves the appearance of skin aging by increasing the expression of ECM proteins in photodamaged skin.

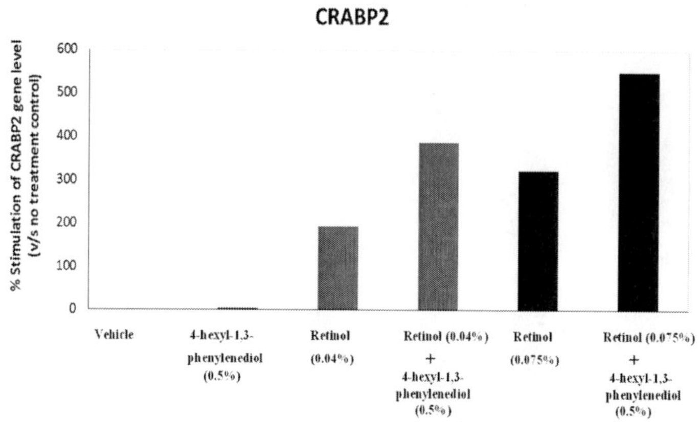

A

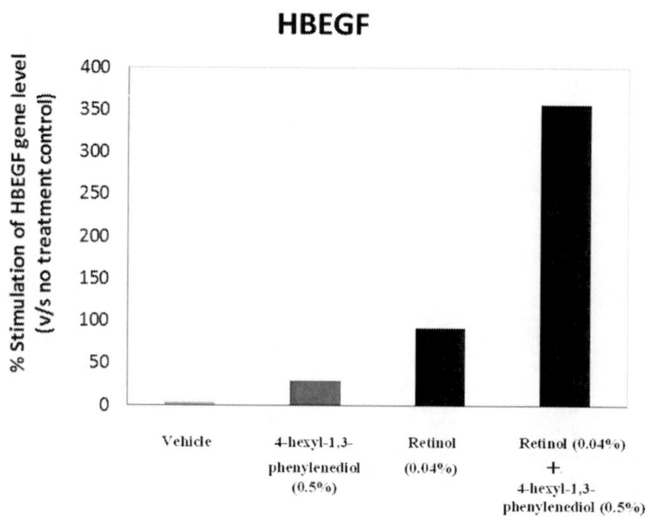

B

Figure 4. (Continued).

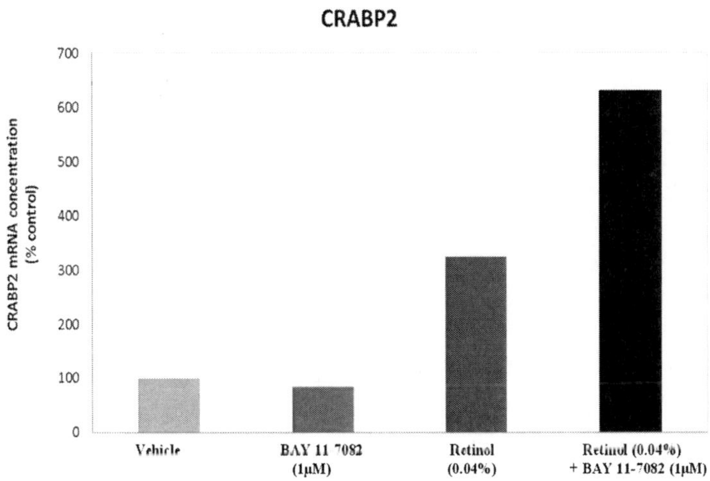

C

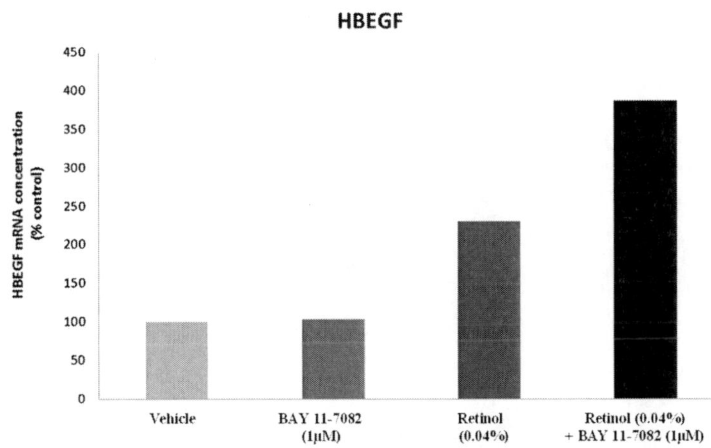

D

Figure 4. Human skin explants were topically treated with the indicated samples for 48 hours, followed by tissue homogenization and RNA isolation from the epidermis. qPCR analysis was performed to measure changes in CRABP2 and HBEGF levels.

Since NF-κB has been shown to inhibit ECM protein expression, it's interesting to speculate that NF-κB inflammation may modulate Retinol anti-aging activity. A link between the efficacy of anti-aging actives and skin inflammation was determined by using Retinol, one of the gold standards in anti-aging, in combination with inhibitors of the NF-κB pathway. Cellular retinoic acid binding protein-II (CRABP2) and Heparin-Binding Epidermal Growth Factor (HBEGF) are known to be reliable indicators of retinol activity in human skin [41, 42].

NF-κB inhibitors synergistically boosted downstream Retinol bioactivity (measured by levels of CRABP2 and HBEGF) in an ex-vivo human skin model, suggesting that blocking inflammation in skin might allow anti-aging actives to work more effectively (Figure 4A-D).

Clinical Studies of Photodaged Skin Involving NF-KB Inhibitors

As people age, they become increasingly concerned with their skin appearance, especially on photo-exposed areas. Clinically, this presents with leathery and yellowish appearance, irregular pigmentation, coarse wrinkles and decreased skin elasticity.

Although there are many topical agents currently marketed for the improvement of photo damaged skin, these products or actives primarily work to address the symptoms of skin aging rather than addressing the biochemical processes which may induce or accelerate skin aging.

Based on the evidence of NF-κB suppressing ECM production in skin and increasing ECM degradation, NF-κB inhibitors may improve photo-damaged skin. Results from 2 recent clinical studies on the NF-κB inhibitor 4-hexyl-1, 3-phenylenediol (HP), support the notion that NF-κB inhibitors do improve photo-damaged skin.

In one study conducted on 65 Asian female subjects, aged 30–40, Fitzpatrick type III and IV in a 12-week, double-blinded study, subjects exhibited significant improvement of photo-damaged skin.

In that study, clinical grading improvements in overall skin lightening, appearance of spots on the cheeks, overall contrast between spots and surrounding skin, and overall pigmentation size, were compared with baseline and placebo [43].

In a second 12-week , placebo-controlled study, subjects who used a 1% HP formulation on their faces saw significant improvements in tone parameters, such as skin radiance, tone evenness, mottled pigmentation, overall skin tone, overall photodamage, as well as crow's feet fine lines, as compared to the placebo (Figure 5) .

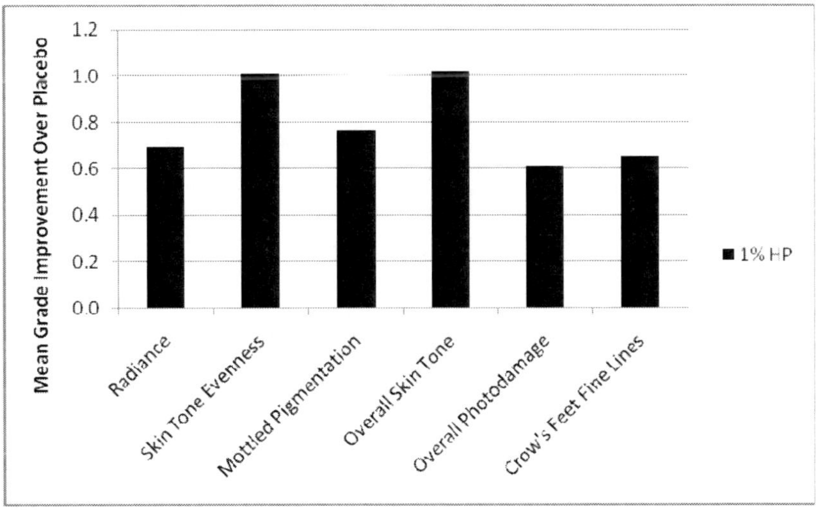

Figure 5. Mean grade improvement of clinical grading in a 12 week anti-aging study demonstrated that topical application of an NF-κB inhibitor significantly improved the appearance of skin aging.

NF-κB Inhibition Boosts the Anti-Aging Efficacy of Retinol

Retinol, a form of Vitamin A, has long been used as a cosmetic skincare ingredient to reduce the signs of aging. Retinol has been shown to increase epidermal thickness, formation of elastin fibers and fibroblast growth potential while decreasing MMP expression [41, 44, 45]. Clinical studies have confirmed that retinol is able to significantly improve many signs of aging in both wrinkles and tone after just four weeks of use [38, 40]. Additionally, the use of 0.1% retinol over the course of an entire year showed continued and significant improvement in treating the appearance of facial skin aging [2].

In another study, after 12 weeks of treatment with either 0.1% retinol or 0.1% retinol and 1% HP, clinical grading showed significant improvement in six separate aging parameters as compared to the placebo control (Figure 6). In all of these signs of aging, the addition of 4-hexyl-1,3-phenylenediol led to a further improvement over retinol alone.

Taken together, these results collectively demonstrate that NF-κB can regulate the age dependent decreased ECM production that contributes to aging. Furthermore, the NF-κB repression of ECM protein expression also appears to modulate the efficacy of anti-aging ingredients that work through inducing ECM expression, suggesting that combinations of NF-κB inhibitors and anti-aging actives may be an effective dual treatment to improve photo-damaged skin.

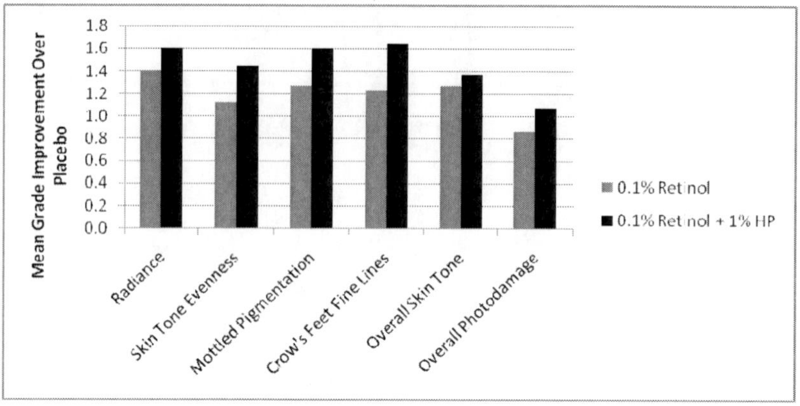

Figure 6. Mean improvement of clinical grading in a 12 week anti-aging study demonstrated that topical combination of Retinol with a NF-κB inhibitor boosted the anti-aging efficacy of Retinol alone.

Conclusion

Skin is a crucial interface that protects the body from environmental insults and performs multiple complex functions, including providing an epithelial barrier, homeostasis, sensory capabilities and immunological protection. However, the skin is constantly under stress from both natural intrinsic factors and environmental extrinsic factors that adversely affect skin health by decreasing skin cell populations and reducing the connective tissue fibres (collagen, elastin, etc.) of the supporting stroma. The cumulative damage to our skin from these environmental aggressors, which include UV radiation and atmospheric pollutants, increases with age, and can result in chronic inflammation and premature aging. Since UV from the sun is continually bombarding our skin, it is constantly under stress, resulting in inflammation. Although some of this inflammation is necessary to maintain and repair the skin, much of it can be associated with long-term photodamage and premature signs of skin aging. While some of these signs may be relieved by taking precautions to minimise exposure to UV, it is near impossible to avoid the damaging effects of UV in their entirety. Furthermore NF-κB inhibition has been reported to induce epidermal proliferation which suggests that NF-κB may regulate multiple epidermal targets of photo-aging as is shown in Figure 7. It is interesting to speculate that inflammation may shunt epidermal keratinocytes from a 'healthy state,' characterized by proliferation and ECM protein expression, to an 'aged state,' characterized by decreased proliferation, decreased ECM production and increased ECM degradation, through the activation of NF-κB. Further speculating, the inflammation process initiated by activation of NF-κB may deprive the cells of energy needed for cell proliferation and shunt cell behaviour instead to inducing inflammatory protein expression. By inhibiting a major pathway responsible for the inflammatory response in the skin and for the loss of matrix proteins, NF-κB inhibitors have been shown to improve several of the signs of photoaged skin.

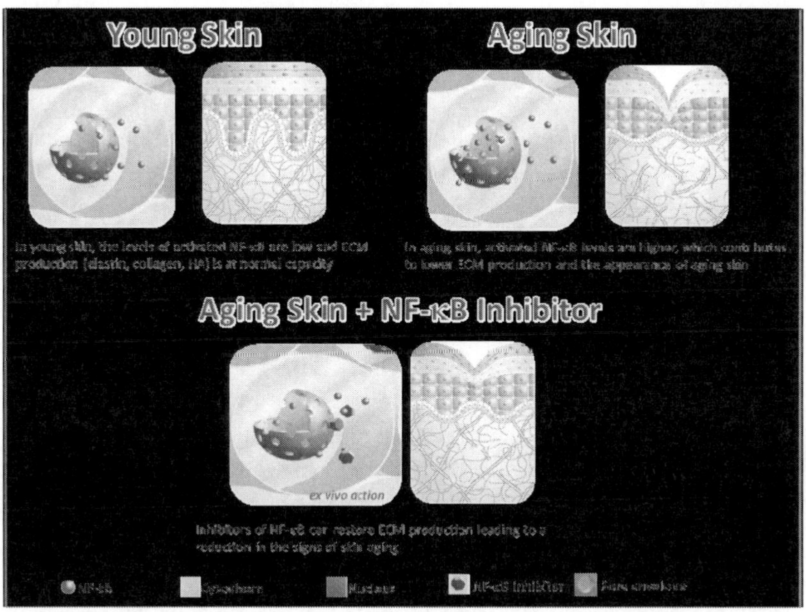

Figure 7. A schematic representation of the proposed effects of NF-κB activation on skin aging and how inhibitors of NF-κB can lead to an improvement in the signs of skin aging.

In addition, NF-κB inhibitors such as 4-hexyl-1,3-phenylenediol appear to increase the effectiveness of other anti-aging actives such as retinol by increasing its bioactivity and resulting in an increased clinical anti-aging efficacy. Taken together, NF-κB inhibitors such, 4-hexyl-1,3-phenylenediol demonstrate great potential as a dermatological tool that can mitigate the signs of premature aging [3] in patients.

References

[1] Scharffetter-Kochanek K, Brenneisen P, Wenk J et al. Photoaging of the skin from phenotype to mechanisms. *Exp. Gerontol.* 2000; 35: 307-16.

[2] Lavker RM. Structural alterations in exposed and unexposed aged skin. *J. Invest. Dermatol.* 1979; 73: 59-66.

[3] Lavker RM, Gerberick GF, Veres D et al. Cumulative effects from repeated exposures to suberythemal doses of UVB and UVA in human skin. *J. Am. Acad. Dermatol.* 1995; 32: 53-62.

[4] Uitto J. The role of elastin and collagen in cutaneous aging: intrinsic aging versus photoexposure. *J. Drugs Dermatol.* 2008; 7: s12-6.

[5] Christensen K, Iachina M, Rexbye H et al. "Looking old for your age": genetics and mortality. *Epidemiology* 2004; 15: 251-2.

[6] Guyuron B, Rowe DJ, Weinfeld AB et al. Factors contributing to the facial aging of identical twins. *Plast Reconstr Surg* 2009; 123: 1321-31.

[7] Fisher GJ, Kang S, Varani J et al. Mechanisms of photoaging and chronological skin aging. *Arch. Dermatol.* 2002; 138: 1462-70.

[8] Jenkins G. Molecular mechanisms of skin ageing. *Mech. Ageing. Dev.* 2002; 123: 801-10.

[9] Fligiel SE, Varani J, Datta SC et al. Collagen degradation in aged/photodamaged skin in vivo and after exposure to matrix metalloproteinase-1 in vitro. *J. Invest. Dermatol.* 2003; 120: 842-8.

[10] Kligman LH, Akin FJ, Kligman AM. The contributions of UVA and UVB to connective tissue damage in hairless mice. *J. Invest. Dermatol.* 1985; 84: 272-6.

[11] Chung JH, Seo JY, Lee MK et al. Ultraviolet modulation of human macrophage metalloelastase in human skin in vivo. *J. Invest. Dermatol.* 2002; 119: 507-12.

[12] Fisher GJ, Datta SC, Talwar HS et al. Molecular basis of sun-induced premature skin ageing and retinoid antagonism. *Nature* 1996; 379: 335-9.

[13] Fisher GJ, Wang ZQ, Datta SC et al. Pathophysiology of premature skin aging induced by ultraviolet light. *N. Engl. J. Med.* 1997; 337: 1419-28.

[14] Li N, Sioutas C, Cho A et al. Ultrafine particulate pollutants induce oxidative stress and mitochondrial damage. *Environ. Health Perspect* 2003; 111: 455-60.

[15] Lademann J, Schaefer H, Otberg N et al. [Penetration of microparticles into human skin]. *Hautarzt* 2004; 55: 1117-9.

[16] Donaldson K, Tran L, Jimenez LA et al. Combustion-derived nanoparticles: a review of their toxicology following inhalation exposure. *Part Fibre. Toxicol.* 2005; 2: 10.

[17] Wan R, Mo Y, Zhang X et al. Matrix metalloproteinase-2 and -9 are induced differently by metal nanoparticles in human monocytes: The role of oxidative stress and protein tyrosine kinase activation. *Toxicol. Appl. Pharmacol.* 2008; 233: 276-85.

[18] Vierkotter A, Schikowski T, Ranft U et al. Airborne particle exposure and extrinsic skin aging. *J. Invest. Dermatol.*; 130: 2719-26.

[19] Valacchi G, Pagnin E, Okamoto T et al. Induction of stress proteins and MMP-9 by 0.8 ppm of ozone in murine skin. *Biochem. Biophys. Res. Commun* 2003; 305: 741-6.

[20] Solly S. Clinical Lectures ON PARALYSIS. *The Lancet* 1856; 68: 641-3.

[21] Lahmann C, Bergemann J, Harrison G et al. Matrix metalloproteinase-1 and skin ageing in smokers. *Lancet* 2001; 357: 935-6.

[22] Yin L, Morita A, Tsuji T. Alterations of extracellular matrix induced by tobacco smoke extract. *Arch. Dermatol. Res.* 2000; 292: 188-94.

[23] Doshi DN, Hanneman KK, Cooper KD. Smoking and skin aging in identical twins. *Arch. Dermatol.* 2007; 143: 1543-6.

[24] Sen R, Baltimore D. Inducibility of kappa immunoglobulin enhancer-binding protein Nf-kappa B by a posttranslational mechanism. *Cell* 1986; 47: 921-8.

[25] Karin M. Nuclear factor-kappaB in cancer development and progression. *Nature* 2006; 441: 431-6.

[26] Karin M, Ben-Neriah Y. Phosphorylation meets ubiquitination: the control of NF-[kappa]B activity. *Annu Rev Immunol* 2000; 18: 621-63.

[27] Baeuerle PA, Baltimore D. NF-kappa B: ten years after. *Cell* 1996; 87: 13-20.

[28] Baeuerle PA, Baichwal VR. NF-kappa B as a frequent target for immunosuppressive and anti-inflammatory molecules. *Adv. Immunol.* 1997; 65: 111-37.

[29] Lu Y, Fukuda K, Li Q et al. Role of nuclear factor-kappaB in interleukin-1-induced collagen degradation by corneal fibroblasts. *Exp. Eye Res.* 2006; 83: 560-8.

[30] Okamoto T, Sakurada S, Yang JP et al. Regulation of NF-kappa B and disease control: identification of a novel serine kinase and thioredoxin as effectors for signal transduction pathway for NF-kappa B activation. *Curr. Top Cell Regul.* 1997; 35: 149-61.

[31] Pahl HL. Activators and target genes of Rel/NF-kappaB transcription factors. *Oncogene* 1999; 18: 6853-66.

[32] Bowie A, O'Neill LA. The interleukin-1 receptor/Toll-like receptor superfamily: signal generators for pro-inflammatory interleukins and microbial products. *J. Leukoc. Biol.* 2000; 67: 508-14.

[33] Baumann L. *Cosmetic dermatology: principles and practice.* New York: McGraw-Hill, 2002.

[34] Habraken Y, Piette J. NF-kappaB activation by double-strand breaks. *Biochem. Pharmacol.* 2006; 72: 1132-41.

[35] Tanaka K, Hasegawa J, Asamitsu K et al. Prevention of the ultraviolet B-mediated skin photoaging by a nuclear factor kappaB inhibitor, parthenolide. *J. Pharmacol. Exp. Ther.* 2005; 315: 624-30.

[36] Helenius M, Kyrylenko S, Vehvilainen P et al. Characterization of aging-associated up-regulation of constitutive nuclear factor-kappa B binding activity. *Antioxid. Redox. Signal.* 2001; 3: 147-56.

[37] Spencer NF, Poynter ME, Im SY et al. Constitutive activation of NF-kappa B in an animal model of aging. *Int Immunol* 1997; 9: 1581-8.

[38] Tucker-Samaras SF, Jared. Poster Abstracts. *Journal of American Academy of Dermatology 69th Annual Meeting* 2011; 64: A4.

[39] Bigot N, Beauchef G, Hervieu M et al. NF-kappaB Accumulation Associated with COL1A1 Transactivators Defects during Chronological Aging Represses Type I Collagen Expression through a -112/-61-bp Region of the COL1A1 Promoter in Human Skin Fibroblasts. *J. Invest. Dermatol.*

[40] Southall MDl, james; fantasia, jared; tucker-samaras, samatha; oddos, thierry. 4-Hexyl-1,3-phenylenediol, an NF-Î°B inhibitor, improves photodamaged skin and clinical signs of aging in a double-blinded, randomized controlled trial. *Poster Abstracts American Academy of Dermatology 72nd Annual Meeting* 2014; 70: AB153.

[41] Kang S, Duell EA, Fisher GJ et al. Application of retinol to human skin in vivo induces epidermal hyperplasia and cellular retinoid binding

proteins characteristic of retinoic acid but without measurable retinoic acid levels or irritation. *J. Invest. Dermatol.* 1995; 105: 549-56.

[42] Bellemere G, Stamatas GN, Bruere V et al. Antiaging action of retinol: from molecular to clinical. *Skin Pharmacol. Physiol.* 2009; 22: 200-9.

[43] Won YK, Loy CJ, Randhawa M et al. Clinical efficacy and safety of 4-hexyl-1,3-phenylenediol for improving skin hyperpigmentation. *Arch. Dermatol. Res.* 2014; 306: 455-65.

[44] Rossetti D, Kielmanowicz MG, Vigodman S et al. A novel anti-ageing mechanism for retinol: induction of dermal elastin synthesis and elastin fibre formation. *Int. J. Cosmet. Sci.*; 33: 62-9.

[45] Varani J, Warner RL, Gharaee-Kermani M et al. Vitamin A antagonizes decreased cell growth and elevated collagen-degrading matrix metalloproteinases and stimulates collagen accumulation in naturally aged human skin. *J. Invest. Dermatol.* 2000; 114: 480-6.

1. Spencer NF, Poynter ME, Im SY, Daynes RA (1997) Constitutive activation of NF-kappa B in an animal model of aging. Int Immunol 9: 1581-1588.
2. Randhawa M, Rossetti D, Leyden JJ, Fantasia J, Zeichner J, et al. One-year Topical Stabilized Retinol Treatment Improves Photodamaged Skin in a Double-blind, Vehicle-controlled Trial. J Drugs Dermatol 14: 271-276.
3. Kaur SK, M.; Fantasia, J.; Oddos, T.; Bigot, N.; Galera, P.; Tucker-Samaras, S.; Leyden, J.J.; and Southall, M.D. (2015) 4-Hexyl-1,3-phenylenediol, an NF-kB inhibitor, improves photodamaged skin and clinical signs of ageing in a double-blinded, randomised controlled trial. British Journal of Dermatology: n/a-n/a.

In: Skin Aging and Photoaging
Editor: Emanuel Graham
ISBN: 978-1-63482-907-6

Chapter 5

Aging Effects on the Physiology of the Stratum Corneum

***Elise Boireau-Adamezyk*[1,2], *Arlette Baillet-Guffroy*[1] *and Georgios N Stamatas*[2]**
[1]Université Paris Sud 11, EA 4041, Châtenay-Malabry, France
[2]Johnson & Johnson Santé Beauté France, Issy-les-Moulineaux, France

Abstract

The advent of non-invasive methods has enabled the study of skin physiology *in vivo*. A wealth of information can thus be acquired about the effects of intrinsic and extrinsic aging, also referred to as chronological aging and photoaging correspondingly, on skin structure, function, and composition. While a lot of work so far has focused on the effects of aging on skin appearance, few studies have dealt with the aging-related changes of the skin barrier and more specifically on the physiology of the epidermal layer that provides most of the barrier function, i.e. the Stratum Corneum (SC). The characteristic structure and composition of this upper part of the human skin confers a veritable barrier to the penetration of external irritants as well as excessive loss of internal water which could lead to dehydration. In the present chapter we will review the relevant methods, the physiological structure and function of the SC, as well as the effects of intrinsic and extrinsic aging on these parameters.

Introduction

The skin is a sensory organ and a biofactory for the synthesis, processing, and metabolism of a wide range of structural proteins, glycans, and lipids [1] fulfilling all the requirements of a classic endocrine organ [2, 3]. The role of the skin is to protect the organism from water loss, temperature change, radiation, and trauma. The important role of the barrier function resides primarily on the upper-most layer of the epidermis, the SC. Non-invasive methods involving probes that can come in contact with the SC can be used to determine the physiological structure and function of the SC *in vivo*. Aging is a progressive process involving reduction in optimal function and renewal capacity of the whole organism [4]. It results in cellular attrition and senescence, eventually terminating by decreased viability and death. It is orchestrated by a genetic program but is also affected by cumulative environmental and endogenous insults that take place throughout the organism's lifespan. The causes of chronological aging are less clear than those of the second type of aging, so called extrinsic aging or photoaging. Photoaged skin is the result of exposure to environmental elements in particular UV radiation, superimposed to chronological skin aging. It sometimes leads to prematurely aged appearance even in young people and is linked to immune suppression. Most of facial aging can be attributed to sun exposure [5]. While some sun exposure is necessary for the production of vitamin D, excessive exposure can lead to tissue damage. Compared to the dermis, little is known about the effects of aging on the epidermis and more specifically on the SC.

The Structure of the Epidermis

The epidermis is the outer, non-vascularized, stratified epithelium, that measures 5 to 100 μm in thickness (although it can reach 600 μm or more on the palms and soles) [6]. It is composed of several distinct cell populations, primarily keratinocytes (90% of the epidermis), melanocytes, and immune cells (Langerhan's cells) [7]. The epidermis is arranged in four layers: underneath the SC one finds sequentially the Stratum Granulosum (SG), the Stratum Spinosum (SS), and the Stratum Basale (SB). In the palms and the soles there is also the Stratum Lucidum, which consists of flattened cells with no nuclei. The epidermis fulfills two main functions due to its structure and metabolism: it protects the skin from external insults and it maintains the hydration of internal tissues [8]. Both functions are realized primarily by the SC, the outer most layer of the epidermis [9].

The keratinocytes originate from dividing cells at the SB, which is in contact with the basement membrane defining the Dermal-Epidermal Junction (DEJ). These cells continue to differentiate as they move from the basal layer to the SC. As the keratinocytes move toward the skin surface, they produce the definitive skin cell protein, keratin, as well as lipids. Their shape changes as they mature. The flattened cell bodies of dead keratinocytes are called corneocytes and they are covered by a highly cross-linked and cornified envelope [10]. The corneocytes provide the barrier against environmental insults. The strength of the epidermal barrier function is inversely related to the rate of Trans-Epidermal Water Loss (TEWL) [11]. The SC contains about 60% proteins, 20% water, and 20% lipids [7, 12]. The efficacy of the water barrier also depends on the SC lipid composition [9] is comprised of cholesterol, ceramides, and long-chain free fatty acids [7, 9]. Both lamellar and lateral lipid organizations contribute to the quality of the barrier function.

Thanks to the SC structure and composition, the water content of the viable portion of the epidermis is maintained at about 70% [13] and decreases toward the skin surface to about 20% w/w. This decrease begins to be observable at the juncture between the SG and the SC [13]. Intercellular lipids, as well as the Natural Moisturizing Factors (NMF), organic acids, and inorganic ions, impact the water-holding capacity of the SC [10]. Several less abundant components in the SC also contribute to maintaining skin hydration, such as Hyaluronic Acid (HA) [14] and glycerol [15]. Moreover, below the SC, aquaporin-3 at the surface of keratinocytes contribute to the water mass balance in the skin [16].

The SG contains flattened, polyhedral non-dividing keratinocytes producing granules of a protein called keratinohyalin. The size and the number of these granules increase as the cell nuclei gradually degenerate leading to cell death. These cells flatten as dividing cells underneath them progressively push them toward the skin surface.

The SS contains irregular polyhedral keratinocytes and Langerhan's cells. The Langerhan's cells are bone marrow-derived sentinel cells of the immune system. They function as antigen-presenting cells of the skin playing a role in immunological reactions such as allergic contact dermatitis. In the SS the cell division capacity is limited.

The SB is also known as the Stratum Germinatum. It is a single layer of cells attached to the basement membrane at the DEJ that separates the epidermis from the dermis. Moreover the basal keratinocytes are situated in the SB and will migrate toward the skin surface. Two other types of cells are found within this layer: Merkel cells (neuroendocrine cells responsible for the transmission of touch sensation through the cutaneous nerves) and melanocytes.

Non-Invasive Methods

Age related changes can be measured by different methods: electric, spectroscopic, chromatographic methods, and imaging applied on biopsy samples or *in vivo*. As it is best to study the tissue in its native state, we will focus on non-invasive methods that are adapted to be used *in vivo*.

Electric-Based Methods

These methods indirectly assess the SC water content by measuring the skin electrical proprieties (impedance, capacitance, and conductance) that depend on the amount of water in the SC. The Corneometer for example measures the ability of the skin to store charges as an electrical capacitor, a property called cutaneous capacitance [17]. The value varies as a function of the water content inside the SC: the more hydrated the SC is, the easier the electric current can flow through the top layers of the epidermis due to the higher ionic mobility in an aqueous environment. Although they are very easy to use, these electric methods have some limitations partially due to the skin lipids. Lipids can prevent the electric flow to pass through, decreasing the skin conductance values and increasing the measured skin capacitance. The concentration of total ionic species may also interfere with the electric conductivity of the skin.

The quality of the SC barrier function can be assessed by the measurement of the rate of TEWL through the SC. When the body is at rest, there is a constant value of in-and-out movement of water resulting in a mass balance equilibrium. Another way to measure the water barrier function is to measure the skin moisture content during a sorption/desorption test [18].

Spectroscopic Methods

All *in vivo* spectroscopic methods rely on the interactions of light with the components of the tissue under investigation.

Diffuse reflectance spectroscopy (DRS) [19] is used to determine the apparent concentration of absorbing molecular species in the UV wavelength called chromophores. In the skin these include melanin, oxygenated hemoglobin, and deoxygenated hemoglobin. The spectra obtained from the tissues have spectral characteristics of these chromophores [20].

Fourier Transform–Near Infrared (FT-NIR) and Mid Infrared (FT-MIR) [21] spectroscopies are based on energy absorption due to molecular bond vibrations. The frequency at which energy is absorbed is characteristic of one kind of the chemical bonds in the structure being analyzed. For example methyl, ethyl, carboxyl groups in their microenvironment can be studied. However, energy absorption of water molecules in the NIR range is very strong and it is difficult to obtain information about other molecular species. It is therefore beneficial to limit the sampling volume to the most superficial layers of the SC that contains about 20% of water. To sample only the superficial layers of the skin it is necessary to use a dispositive called Attenuated Total Reflectance (ATR) crystal [20]. Using this type of probe only the very superficial part of the skin is studied (1 to 2 μm depending on the wavelength). ATR-FTIR spectra are obtained providing detailed vibrational information on molecular composition and molecular structure. Good and reliable measurements of water and skin lipids are obtained, whether they come from sebaceous glands or the SC. Surface information about the lipid organization with the FTIR technique can be obtained. Tissue absorption rates of an active compound [22] can also be studied by the rate of reduction of its surface concentration.

Raman spectroscopy [23] is another vibrational method that is a well-adapted tool for studying *in vivo* the supramolecular organization and biochemical composition of the SC. *In vivo* confocal Raman spectroscopy is able to measure spectra at specific depths from the skin surface down to 100–200 μm [24, 25]. The penetration depth is limited by multiple scattering events, the numerical aperture of the objective, and the photon absorption in the tissue. Structural and organizational information of molecular bonds have characteristic signatures in Raman spectroscopy. It is possible to deduce the nature and the structure of a molecule in free or bonded forms and also the interaction with its environment [26]. This method can be used to collect information about the quality of the SC barrier function, the hydration state of the SC, and the SC thickness. It can also be used to study the penetration of an active substance and its concentration distribution through the SC.

Fluorescence spectroscopy has been used to study skin physiology [27–39]. It has been shown that dry keratins fluoresce brighter than when hydrated. The epidermal cell proliferation rate has been related to the signal of tryptophan moieties (excitation maximum at 295 nm and emission maximum at 345 nm) [30]. It has been shown that when the rate of the epidermal cell proliferation increases, the tryptophan signal also increases [27]. Biochemical stimulation [29] or exposure to UV radiation [27] may induce tryptophan fluorescence. The tryptophan fluorescence intensity decreases with aging reflecting the decreased capacity of epidermal cells to proliferate.

Imaging Methods

Ordinary visible light microscopy can be used to get information about the micro relief line density and patterns, pore size, and melanin distribution.

The spectroscopic adaptation of imaging (e.g. fluorescence or spectral imaging) can be used to examine the spatial distribution and variation of molecular concentrations of interest. This is an extension of the single point information that it is otherwise obtained by regular spectroscopy.

Spectral imaging can be used to identify and quantify chromophores or molecular species due to their characteristic absorption bands [40, 41]. The skin depth probed depends on the absorption and scattering proprieties of the skin and on the wavelength of the light source.

The chemical information obtained by Raman spectroscopy can be combined with the spatial distribution in Raman microscopy. Raman spectral imaging at the cellular level has been used to get information relating to apoptosis, cell growth and differentiation, and product-cell interaction [42].

In vivo reflectance Confocal Microscopy (RCM) is used to capture light that has gone through a single scattering event in the tissue [43]. The amount of collected light is limited by the numerical aperture of the objective and photon absorption. The laser source is scanned in a horizontal plane that optically transverses the tissue. At a cellular level architectural details that can be evaluated including epidermal thickness [44, 45], keratinocyte disorder with aging [46, 47], the compaction of keratin in the SC, the effects of aging on melanocytes, the distribution of melanosomes inside melanocytes, melanin production, and changes in the nuclei.

Optical Coherence Tomography (OCT) [43–45, 48–53] is a non-invasive imaging method generating vertical cross-sectional images of the skin capable to present morphological features of the epidermal and papillary dermis. The axial resolution (about 5 μm) and the quality of image are comparable to RCM. The recorded signal depends on the optical proprieties of the skin and primarily scattering. This method involves a fiber optic Michelson interferometer with a low coherence length broadband light source as IR [53, 54]. OCT is not capable to routinely differentiate between the SC and the viable epidermis. The determination of the mean skin thickness is in agreement with cryostat-histology, considered as the gold standerd to assess the epidermal thickness [55].

The phenomenon of two-photon microscopy [56] occurs when two photons with the same wavelength interact and their energy recombines resulting in a single photon that has double their frequency (or equivalently half their wavelength). A pulsed laser is used with a high repetition rate (MHz range) and with very short pulses: 10^{-15}s. The laser light (typically in NIR) excites the UV fluorescing molecular species in the skin. It is able to propagate deep into the skin as the absorption and the scattering coefficients are minimal.

Chromatographic Methods

Chromatographic methods, including gas and liquid chromatography are able to provide molecular information for distinct molecular groups, such as lipid species to result in lipid profiles [57]. In general, liquid chromatography (normal phase or reverse phase) or gas chromatography are used with a detection system, which can be the evaporative light scattering detector or charged aerosol detector (Corona) [58] for quantitative studies or High Resolution Mass Spectroscopy (HR-MS^n) for qualitative studies. Skin surface lipids (also named hydrolipidic film) and SC lipids can be acquired with minimally invasive methods such as absorbing papers for the first type and tape-stripping or solvent extraction for the second. These analytical techniques are particularly useful for generating lipid profiles [59] because of the complexity of the hydrolipidic film lipid or SC lipid composition. The importance of ceramides sub-classes and their length and unsaturated chains on compactness of lipid edifices has been clearly shown. Only the chromatographic methods can give qualitative and quantitative information about these compositions [60, 61]. This kind of molecular information is very interesting because it can give some explanation of the aging effects on the barrier properties.

Skin Aging

1. Intrinsic (Chronological) Aging

Visual Appearance [62, 63]

The processes involved in wrinkle formation have been discussed by others [64, 65]. Here we will focus on aging effects on the epidermis and more specifically its outer most part, the SC. Skin atrophy is accompanied by an increase in fragility, dryness with pruritus and xerosis with the apparition of a variety of benign neoplasms such as seborrheic keratoses and angiomas. With age the skin becomes more susceptible to irritation [66] and there is a decrease in sensorial perception.

Thickness of the SC and the Viable Epidermis

Some authors found that the total epidermal thickness remains constant with increasing age [67, 68].

Concerning the thickness of the SC histological studies show different results: some observed that the SC thickness does not change with age [69, 70] and some authors found a slight increase [71].

Some studies report that thickness of the viable epidermis tends to decrease [72–74] progressively at a rate that accelerates with age [75]. Indeed, the overall human non-exposed epidermis decreases by ~10-50% between 30 and 80 years old [70, 76] equivalent to 6% per decade [77, 78].

Not only the thickness of the total epidermis decreases but also the resistance to pressure is diminished [74, 79]. These different conclusions can be explained by the small physiological variations and depend on the group of age of interest.

Barrier Function

The skin barrier function is complex. It is primarily located in the SC and is the result of many factors including the composition and the organization of the intercellular lipid cement. The strength of the barrier function depends on the location of the body site of interest [71]. The results published in the literature are sometimes contradictory as the employed method, the population demographics, and/or the skin site may be different.

The most common method to evaluate the quality of the skin barrier function is by measuring the TEWL.

In the published literature one finds different results concerning the evolution of the barrier function with aging: some studies demonstrated no change in TEWL rates with aging [80, 81] indicating that the barrier function is not altered significantly with aging [81–83]. Other studies show that the barrier function slightly improves with aging [71, 10, 84–86]. However, the causes of reduced rate of TEWL of aged epidermis are not known [80].

The barrier function can also be evaluated by the measurement of the penetration rate in the epidermis of exogenous molecules topically applied. In one report caffeine penetration has been proposed as a marker to evaluate the perturbation of the barrier function [87].

Research has been recently focused on the origin of the barrier function at the molecular and supramolecular level. Chromatographic and spectroscopic methods are used to study the age-dependent evolution of the hydrolipidic film and the SC lipid composition and organization.

Although some studies indicate little or no relationship between age and lipid content [88, 89], many authors accept that overall total lipid content decreases in the SC with age [71, 90] by about 30%. This reflects the slower keratinocyte metabolism of the aged skin [91, 92] that results in a decrease in biosynthetic capacity. However, Cua et al., [88] compared lipid composition with small angle X-ray diffraction and they did not find differences between an older and a younger group: relative ratios of each of the major lipid classes (cholesterol, fatty acid and individual ceramide species) are constant throughout life.

Denda et al., [93] showed by High Performance Thin Layer Chromatography (HPTLC) that from puberty to adulthood there is an increase of the ratio of the ceramide1 (or EOS) and ceramide 2 (or NS) to the total sphingolipid amount and a decrease of the ratio ceramide 3 (or NP) and ceramide 6 (or NH) to the total sphingolipid amount (definition of subclasses according to the classification by Rabionet et al., [94]). The ratio of ceramide 2 to the total sphingolipid amount decreases with age and that of ceramide 3 to total sphingolipid increases with age. Moreover, the SC sphingolipid composition depends on the epidermal biosynthesis of sphingolipids that is influenced first by the epidermal proliferative activity [95] and secondly by the presence of hormones. This also suggests that the age-associated decrease in hormone levels may impact the skin barrier function in the elderly [93].

Rogers et al., [91] found by HPTLC that all classes of ceramides decrease by 30% with age on the face, hands, and legs in older subjects (limited to subjects up to 50 years of age). It is most marked for the levels of ceramide species 1-6, on the face and the hand but the percentage ratios of the individual species remained constant. The SC lipid levels also depend on the skin site (face, hands and legs). Ceramide 1 linoleate decreases with age on the leg. This depletion of ceramide 1 linoleate contributes to the formation of an intrinsically weaker SC with an increase of susceptibility to dysfunction of desquamation and xerosis. Age-effects on SC lipids are not limited to ceramides. Rogers et al., [91] and separately our team [71] found that cholesterol decreases on the face, although the percentage ratio of cholesterol to lipid is constant. They also found a decrease in fatty acid levels, but with a constant ratio of fatty acid to lipids [91, 92, 96]. Makrantonaki & Zouboulis showed that the cholesterol content decreases [97] on the cheek with age. Saint Léger et al., found a decrease in sterol esters and triglycerides with age [92] on the lower legs.

The decline in cholesterol, ceramides and free fatty acids content can be attributed to the reduced activities of key rate-limiting enzymes for each of these lipids including serine palmitoyl transferase (SPT), 3-hydroxy-3-methylglutaryl-coenzyme A (HMG-CoA) reductase, and acetyl CoA carboxytase (ACC) [98].

Lipid organization plays a key role in the barrier function [99–101]. Lipids form multilamellar sheets within the intercellular spaces of the SC, the organization of which is essential in maintaining the functionality of the skin as an effective barrier to water loss [102, 103]. Spectroscopic methods are pertinent tools for this purpose. The conformational order is reported to be directly related to the lateral packing [104–106]. Tfayli et al., showed that aging leads to the loosening of the organizational order and a decrease in the ordered inter-molecular structure [107]. In parallel they also showed that with aging there is a decrease of the trans/gauche conformation structures in the alkyl chain of lipids indicating a lower intra-chain order and inducing an increase in the lateral packing disorder [107]. Our team has reported a decrease of the lipid compactness on the exposed arm site and on the protected arm site with aging [71].

Interestingly, Cua et al., [88] and Saint Léger et al., [92] found no relationship between the skin surface lipid content and age except on the ankle, with the older group showing an increase in lipid content. Other authors report that the skin surface lipids at a very old age are similar to those of pre-pubertal children [108]. However, sebum production could be a more complicated process between the young people and the elderly. Sebaceous glands are well developed in neonates but their size tends to change with age [109]. They become smaller a few weeks after birth and they are almost undetectable during childhood [110, 111]. Their size increases again with the adrenarche, develops further with the onset of puberty, reaches its maximum at the 3rd decade of life, remains constant until after menaupose, tends to decrease slowly at the 7th decade [112], and shows no significant change after the 7th decade. As for the keratinocytes, 17β-estradiol progesterone (during menaupose) reduces sebaceous differentiation [113, 114]. The concomitant decrease in the production of androgens may explain the decrease in sebaceous gland synthesis and secretion. Moreover the turnover rate of the sebaceous glands in older skin is reduced compared to young. Other factors such as hormones, gender, and race influence the sebum secretion besides age. Sebum production on the human face has been found to vary with age according to Le Fur et al., [108] However, there is a paradox concerning the aging of facial skin. On the face the volume of the sebaceous glands increases with age but paradoxically their secretory output decreases [109, 111, 115] accompanied by a decrease in the surface lipid levels. Although sebum production declines in old age, the size of the follicular reservoir may not because the sebaceous glands undergo hypertrophy in older individuals [115].

Other factors implied in the barrier function should be considered such as the pH and the calcium gradient.

Skin surface pH is relatively constant from childhood to approximately 70 years of age [77] then rises significantly. This phenomenon is especially pronounced in lower limbs [77] possibly due to impaired circulation [77]. Wilhelm et al., and Zlotogorski also showed that facial skin pH is more alkaline in aged subjects and that regional differences exists among the various areas of the face [83, 116]. Wilhelm et al., found that the forearm has the most alkaline pH and the forehead has the most acidic pH that increases with aging [83].

The role of calcium in lamellar body secretion is well known. Altered calcium gradient in aged epidermis could account for the barrier abnormality [117]. Aging blunts the calcium concentration gradient through the epidermis [117] due to a decrease in the activity of ions pumps, ions channels, and/or ionotropic receptors in aged skin. In aged human epidermis both the internal structure of lamellar bodies, as well as their numbers in the cytosol of granular cells, are similar to those in young subjects. However, variations were evident in the structures of the unsaturated fatty acids. Aged epidermis displays a decrease in secreted lamellar body-derived contents and a failure of these contents to form a continuous series of multilamellar bilayers within the intercellular spaces of SC [80].

Following acute insults, barrier recovery is delayed in aged skin [80, 98, 118]. Functionally the time required to recover from an epidermal wound, for example blistering, increases by about 50% between young and older adults [95, 119]. It takes 3 days in young adults and 6 days in elderly adults to recover from a blistering insult [80]. In young epidermis, barrier abrogation is followed by a repair process that involves: 1) immediate secretion of preformed epidermal lamellar bodies; 2) replenishment of the cytosol with newly formed lamellar bodies and further secretion of lamellar body contents; 3) formation of lamellar bilayers in the SC interstices leading to recovery of the barrier to TEWL within 24 hours.

The aged epidermal permeability barrier is easier to perturb. Older skin seems to absorb topical substances more slowly than young skin [120]. Depending on the compound there may be differences in the rate of percutaneous absorption, which may explain conflicting results concerning the percutaneous absorption [121]. The rate of percutaneous absorption also depends on the body site [90]. Hydrophobic compounds penetrate more easily in areas of the body skin that have a high percentage of skin lipids [90].

SC Water Content

Concerning the effects of aging on the SC water content conflicting reports exist in the literature, either showing that SC water content does not change [83, 122, 85] or that it slightly decreases [7, 8, 71, 75, 124]. The vibrational energy of OH bonds in the water molecule depends on the formation of hydrogen bonds at the local microenvironment. Water molecules that form non-covalent bonds to other compounds have been termed as called "bound" water. Other water molecules form hydrogen bonds with neighboring water molecules in a tetrahedral structure. These molecules are called tetrahedron or bulk water [124–128].

Intrinsic aging does not appear to alter water structure significantly [129]. Gniadecka et al., show that in the epidermis of young skin the water is present mainly in "bound" form [130, 126, 127, 131]. Vyumvuhore et al., distinguished between bound water, weakly bound, and bound water in the SC *ex vivo* using confocal Raman microspectroscopoy [132]. Following that report our group showed in an *in vivo* study that the distribution of the three states of water according to molecular mobility are independent of age [133]. Bulgin & Vinson [134] showed by differential thermal analysis that the bound water represents 34% of the normal SC dry weight that is equal to 80% of the total SC water. The water-holding capacity of the SC depends on the skin site. Egawa & Tagami showed that the SC water content at a depth of 10-30 μm in the forearm skin tends to be lower in older subjects than in younger subjects [135]. On the other hand no difference was found in the much thinner SC of the cheek between different age groups in facial water-holding capacity and skin conductance.

Mechanical Function

The SC water content plays an important role in controlling the activity of the enzymes involved in the corneocyte desquamation. Reduction in the levels of SC water content can lead to altered desquamation and accumulation of corneocytes at the skin surface, resulting in skin surface roughness, scaliness, and flaking that accompany xerosis in aged skin. The corneocytes become larger due to a decreased epidermal turnover rate [121, 136]. They clump together on the surface, the surface becomes rough with a scaly appearance and texture [137]. The increase in corneocytes size that accompanies aging process [138] may compensate for the effects of reduced lipid content.

Vyumvuhore et al., studied the behaviors of the SC components during water desorption, following a drying process using Raman spectroscopy [139]. Mechanical stress of the SC mainly depends on the concentration of the bulk water.

Epidermal Cell Turnover Rate

Keratinocytes generated in the basal layer migrate toward the SC, where they become corneocytes and finally are eliminated at the skin surface. This epidermal cell turnover rate depends on the skin body site and the age.

Epidermal cell turnover rates decrease by about 50% from 20 to 70 years of age, which leads to epidermal atrophy at the histological level and to a thinner epidermis. Even if there is a decrease of the epidermal cell proliferation the number of cells layers remains stable [121]. TGF-β1 could be a potent inhibitor of epidermal growth as this multifunctional cytokine regulates cell proliferation and differentiation, tissue remodeling, and repair. In young and healthy skin, one layer of corneocytes desquamates every day. The whole SC replaces itself in about 15-20 days [10] in young skin in contrast with the elderly SC that may take twice as long, 40-60 days [95, 140]. The decrease in epidermal cell turnover rate may in part explain the decrease in skin barrier function and why the repair process is delayed in the aged [120].

Globally, there is an overall reduction in epidermal cell number [141] with aging in the epidermis. Senescent cells are accumulating in aging human skin.

Decline in the integrity and function of the skin and possibly other tissues, associated with aging, is due it the presence of senescent cells.

Biochemical Composition

Skin aging is accompanied by a decline in the NMF production according to McCallion [8]. The term NMF represents a mix of hygroscopic molecules: free fatty acids, Pyrrolidone Carboxylic Acid (PCA), urea, lactate ions, and sugars. The NMF helps retain water molecules in the SC. In older people the SC of the cheek and the forearm contains more NMF than the SC of young individuals. The increase of the NMF content may be the result of a slower SC turnover rate in aged skin that allows longer time for the proteolysis of the filaggrin to be converted into NMF [10, 15]. The aged epidermis of the forearm contains more free amino acids and more trans-Urocanic acid than the young epidermis. There is a decline with age of the SC urea content [135]. Urea is a component of sweat and contributes to the hydration of the SC. The SC urea content is significantly lower for women > 55 years of age for the upper inner arm site [142]. No age-related differences were detected within the volar forearm site [142].

Age-related changes are not well defined for the SC lactate content, which is another sweat component [135]. Some studies report that it declines with age. The SC lactate content is significantly lower for women > 55 years of age in the upper inner arm site [142]. No age-related differences were detected within the volar forearm site. HA has recently been shown to be present naturally in the epidermis and is considered to be part of the NMF [14]. The decrease of HA in intrinsically aged skin may also play a critical role for other age-related effects, including lower keratinocyte proliferation rate and thinner epidermis [143]. HA is binding to the extracellular space via the protein CD43 [14, 144]. Oh et al., show that the epidermal water content is correlated with both HA and total sulfated Glycose Amino Glycans (tsGAG) [143].

The epidermis possesses an extremely efficient antioxidant system that is superior to most other tissues [145]. This system displays a decrease in efficiency as a function of skin aging [146]. Ascorbic acid levels are lower in the epidermis of both photoaged and aged skin, while α-tocopherol (known as vitamin E) is lower in the epidermis but not in the dermis. Other antioxidant molecules and enzymes such as Cu, Zn, super oxide dismutase (SOD), catalase, and glutathione peroxidase levels also decrease with age [145, 147].

The human epidermis plays a role in the generation of the active form of vitamin D, $1.25(OH)_2D_3$. Besides its role in calcium homeostasis and bone maintenance, vitamin D has been implicated in immune responses, affecting macrophage function and modulating the release of inflammatory cytokines [148, 149]. Therefore, when the synthesis of vitamin D decreases, the immune response is also impaired [150]. Elderly people have reduced serum levels of vitamin D in their diet, which in part may be due to insufficient sun exposure.

Reduced cytokine production [151] and/or downstream reactivity in skin have been associated with aging [152]. Interleukin (IL)-1α and IL-1β are the major keratinocyte cytokines. They are normally expressed in all epidermal cell layers and barrier disruption markedly enhances both IL-1α mRNA and protein levels. In contrast aged epidermis expresses subnormal mRNA and protein levels of certain members of this cytokine family [138, 154].

2. Extrinsic (Photo) Aging

Visual Appearance [109, 155–157]

The term "photoaging" was used for the first time in 1986. It describes the effects of chronic UV light exposure on the skin [158]. Typically, individuals who follow outdoors lifestyles and live in sunny places are expected to have some degree of photoaging. During human life different body skin sites are exposed at varying levels. UV light can cause lipid peroxidation in the SC and DNA damage in the viable epidermis.

Long term effects of sunlight on skin are profound and it is estimated that they account for up to 90% of visible skin aging [159], particularly in people without the natural protection associated with higher levels of melanin content in the skin [160]. Quantitative and qualitative photoaging can remain invisible for decades before clinical signs become evident. The changes induced by chronic sun exposure can occur well before visible signs of chronological aging and depend on skin type, nature of sun exposure (occupational vs recreational), hair style, and dress.

The effects on the skin following exposure to UV radiation include changes in surface texture [161], early appearance of dyschromia and lentigines, increased roughness, and the development of fine rhytides [161].

Thickness of the SC and the Epidermis

Corneocytes of photoaged skin become polymorphic with increasing abnormalities: retention of nuclear remnants and roughening of border edges [121, 162]. The epidermal thickness of exposed skin is modified. Extrinsic aging shows an irregular thickening of the epidermis: [5] the epidermal thickness increases (corresponding to hyperplasia) then decreases (corresponding to severe atrophy). It is unlikely that UV-induced effects play a major role in a decrease of epidermal thickness with age [73].

Some authors found an increase of the SC thickness of the exposed skin site [71]. With respect to UVB-induced erythema the SC thickness appears to be a more efficient shield for photoprotection than either the extent of pigmentation or the total thickness of viable epidermis [163].

Barrier Function

The superposition of photoaging and aging further aggravates barrier abnormality [118]. Skin Surface Lipids (SSL, squalene in particular) which coat the surface of sebaceous gland-enriched skin sites, such as the face, are first-line targets of UV light. Irradiation of squalene with UVB and UVA leads to formation of squalene hydroperoxide [164–166] resulting in oxidative stress. Photoaging is associated with the development of benign and malignant sebaceous tumors often located on the head and neck area [167]. Sebaceous gland hyperplasia develops mainly in ageing facial skin. However, sebaceous glands hyperplasia also occurs in the oral mucosa of elderly person where sunlight is not a relevant issue [109].

SC Water Content

Gniadecka et al., found that photoaged skin has increased levels of SC water content observed by Raman Spectroscopy [129]. This is paradoxal as the aged skin surface is often dry. Boireau et al found using *in vivo* confocal Raman microspectroscopy a decrease of the SC water content on photoaged skin [71]. However, the changes are small.

Biochemical Composition

UV irradiation (<320 nm) converts the epidermal precursor of vitamin D_3 and dehydrocholesterol to previtamin D_3, which subsequently isomerizes to form vitamin D_3. With aging the levels of the epidermal precursor of vitamin D_3 decrease contributing to a decrease in vitamin D_3 production in older populations [168]. This can result in vitamin D3 deficiency in the absence of regular sun exposure [169]. Vitamin A is destroyed by sun exposure.

Following chronic UV exposure the levels of oxidatively modified proteins significantly increase [170, 171]. UV filtration by the SC and the greater antioxidant capacity of the epidermis protect to some extend the nucleated epidermal layers. Remarkably catalase protein and activity levels are naturally present at a very high concentration in human SC and become significantly depleted upon UV exposure *in vivo* [170, 172]. Hellmans et al., [172] showed that catalase levels and activity are strongly affected by UVA but remain unchanged upon UVB exposure. Recovery of the catalase enzyme after UV exposure occurred in 3-4 weeks following an age-depend fashion. Recovery is faster in younger individuals than in older [173].

UV radiation stimulates and activates various cells to produce and release cytokines that may play a significant role in the process of photoaging [174].

Other Triggers of Accelerated Skin Aging

Intrinsic factors including inter-individual variations of genetic and epigenetic mechanisms have been linked to individual differences in the aging process. Manifestations of skin aging vary for different ethnic groups: for example thinning of the epidermis may be different between light and dark complexioned people [175]. Extrinsic factors that affect the aging process, beyond UV radiation and smoking, include air pollution, temperature variations, and lifestyle. Malnutrition may also provoke premature skin aging by causing metabolic disturbance and lack of important proteins, ions, and co-enzymes. A relation between smoking and wrinkling was noted as early as 1876 [176]. In 1972, Daniell showed that smoking has a deleterious effect on the skin and appearance. In an epidemiologic study tobacco smoking has been shown to be one of the most important factors contributing to premature skin aging. Due to photosensitization [177], smokers look older than non-smokers of the same age [178]. From an epidermal viewpoint, smoking increases keratinocyte dysplasia and skin roughness [4]. More generally, unbalanced nutrition, excessive dieting, and stress may provoke premature skin aging.

Conclusion

In this review the main effects of chronological and extrinsic aging on the SC are highlighted, summarized in Table 1. The observed effects depend on the used method, the body skin sites and the groups of age. Intrinsic aging and extrinsic aging lead to visible and non-visible modifications of the epidermal skin at tissue, cellular and molecular level. Some changes are the results of cell senescence, while others are linked to environmental insults such as UV radiation, exposure to temperature extremes or stress. The age-related modifications that are observable macroscopically can be attributed to changes that happen at the molecular, supramolecular, and cellular level.

Table 1.

		Intrinsic aging	**Extrinsic (photo)aging**
STRUCTURE	SC / Epidermal Thickness	SC thickness: Marks [69] and Lock-Andersen et al., [70] reported no change in SC thickness, Boireau et al., [71] showed an increase of the SC thickness. Viable Epidermal thickness: Lavker & Kligman [72] and Lavker [73] and Branchet et al., [74] showed a tendency to decrease of the epidermal thickness with a rate that accelerates with aging. The resistance to pressure is also diminished [74, 79]. Epidermal thickness: El-Domyati et al., [67] and Whitton & Everall. [68] found a constant epidermal thickness with aging.	Exposed epidermal thickness: Gilchrest [5] reported an irregular thickening of the epidermis, increase and decrease of the thickness. For Lavker [73], UV-induced effects play a major role in the decrease of epidermal thickness with age. Boireau et al., [71] found an increase of the SC thickness with aging of the exposed skin site.
FUNCTION	Barrier Function	TEWL: Ghadially et al., [80] and Roskos & Guy [81] reported no change in TEWL rates with aging; the SC barrier function is not altered significantly. Boireau et al., [71], Tagami [10], Berardesca & Maibach [84], Cua et al., [85], Kobayashi & Tagami [86] found that the SC barrier function evolves with aging. Lipid content: Cua et al. [88] and Schreiner et al. [89] showed no relationship between age and lipid content, Boireau et al., [71] and Roskos & Maibach [90] reported a decrease of the SC lipid content with aging.	Aggravation of the barrier abnormality with superimposition of both effects (intrinsic and extrinsic aging) showed by Reed et al. [118]

		Intrinsic aging	Extrinsic (photo)aging
		Cua et al., [88] reported that the cholesterol, fatty acid and ceramides contents are constant throughout life. Rogers et al., [91], Boireau et al., [71] and Makrantonaki & Zouboulis [97] showed the cholesterol content decreases on the face but its percentage is constant throughout life. Rogers et al., [91], Saint Léger et al., [92] and Roskos [96] showed that the percentage of fatty acid is constant with aging. Rogers et al., [91] showed that the ceramide content decreases by 30% with aging on the face, hands and legs. Denda et al., [93] found that according to the time of life, some subclasses of ceramides increase, and some subclasses of ceramides decrease. Lipid structure: Aging is accompanied to the loosening of the organizational order and a decrease in the ordered inter-molecular structure according to Tfayli et al. [107] There is also a decrease of the trans/gauche conformation structures in the alkyl chain of lipids in the older skin indicating a lower intra-chain order and inducing an increase in the lateral packing disorder [107]. According to Boireau et al., [71] there is a decrease of the lipid compactness on the exposed arm site and on the protected arm site with aging.	

Table 1. (Continued)

		Intrinsic aging	Extrinsic (photo)aging
		Skin Surface lipids: Increase of the SSL content with age except on the ankle according to Cua et al., [88] and Saint Léger et al. [92] Sebaceous glands: The size of sebaceous glands varies with aging. Le Fur et al., [108] showed that the level of sebaceous glands in the on the face of elderly is similar to those of pubertal children. In aged skin the turnover of the sebaceous glands is slowed down compared to the young skin. Sebum: The sebum production declines with age pH: According to Waller & Maibach [77] the pH is constant until 70 years old and then rises, except on facial skin where the pH is more alkaline in aged subjects. Calcium: According to Denda et al., [117] the altered calcium gradient with aging accounts for the barrier abnormality. Barrier recovery: Ghadially et al., [80] showed that it takes 3 days in young population to recover the barrier and 6 days in old population. Topical substances are consequently absorbed more slowly in old people than young people.	

		Intrinsic aging	**Extrinsic (photo)aging**
	SC water content	Eisner et al., [122], Wilhelm et al., [83] and Cua et al., [85] reported no change of the global SC water content with age while Jackson et al. [7], McCallion & Po [8], Harvell & Maibach [75], Walrafen [124] and Boireau et al., [71] reported a slightly decrease of the SC water content with age. According to Gniadecka et al., [129] there is no alteration of the water structure with aging.	Increase of the SC water content with age, and paradoxally aged skin surface is often dry and weathered according to Gniadecka et al. [129] No alterations of the water structure [129]. Boireau et al., [71] found a decrease of the SC water content on the exposed arm site with aging
	Mechanical	The corneocytes become bigger due to a decreased epidermal turnover leading to roughness of the skin [121, 136].	The corneocytes become polymorphic with roughening of border edges [121,162].
	Cellular proliferation	The epidermal cell proliferation decreases by about 50% from 20 to 70 years old but number of cells remain stable [121]. Tagami [10] found that the SC is replaced by 15-20 days in young skin, while Grove & Kligman [95] and Baker & Blair [140] found that the SC is replaced in 40-60 in old skin.	The response to chronic UV exposure depends to the individual's skin type. Changes in cell number are also prominent in sun-exposed skin beginning in childhood.
COMPOSITION	Biochemical composition	NMF: McCallion & Po [8] showed that there is a decline in NMF production. Elderly skin of the cheek and the forearm contain more NMF than in the young skin. Decline of urea content according to Egawa & Tagami [135].	Vitamin: Decrease of vitamin D3 in older population, destruction of vitamin A by sun exposure [168].

Table 1. (Continued)

		Intrinsic aging	Extrinsic (photo)aging
		Even if the decline of the SC lactate content with age is not so well-defined, there is a significantly lower lactate content for women 55 years old and over in the upper inner arm site according to Wu & Kilpatrick-Liverman [142] Decrease of hyaluronic acid content according to Oh et al., [143] Decrease of efficiency of antioxidant activity [146]	

References

[1] Chuong, C. M. et al., What is the 'true' function of skin? *Exp. Dermatol.* 11, 159–187 (2002).

[2] Zouboulis, C. C. Human Skin: An Independent Peripheral Endocrine Organ. *Horm. Res.* 54, 230–242 (2000).

[3] Zouboulis, C. The human skin as a hormone target and an endocrine gland. *Horm. Athens Greece* 3, 9–26 (2003).

[4] Yaar, M., Eller, M. S. & Gilchrest, B. A. Fifty Years of Skin Aging. *J. Investig. Dermatol. Symp. Proc.* 7, 51–58 (2002).

[5] Gilchrest, B. A. Skin aging and photoaging: An overview. *J. Am. Acad. Dermatol.* 21, 610–613 (1989).

[6] Tobin, D. J. Biochemistry of human skin—our brain on the outside. *Chem. Soc. Rev.* 35, 52–67 (2006).

[7] Jackson, S. M., Williams, M. L., Feingold, K. R. & Elias, P. M. Pathobiology of the stratum corneum. *West. J. Med.* 158, 279–285 (1993).

[8] McCallion, R. & Po, A. L. W. Dry and photo–aged skin:and manifestations management. *J. Clin. Pharm. Ther.* 18, 15–32 (1993).

[9] Elias, P. M. Stratum corneum architecture, metabolic activity and interactivity with subjacent cell layers. *Exp. Dermatol.* 5, 191–201 (1996).

[10] Tagami, H. Functional characteristics of the stratum corneum in photoaged skin in comparison with those found in intrinsic aging. *Arch. Dermatol. Res.* 300, 1–6 (2007).

[11] Elias, P. M. Stratum Corneum Defensive Functions: An Integrated View. *J. Gen. Intern. Med.* 20, 183–200 (2005).

[12] Mathias, C. G. T. & Maibach, H. I. Perspectives in Occupational Dermatology. *West. J. Med.* 137, 486–492 (1982).

[13] Caspers, P. J., Lucassen, G. W. & Puppels, G. J. Combined In Vivo Confocal Raman Spectroscopy and Confocal Microscopy of Human Skin. *Biophys. J.* 85, 572–580 (2003).

[14] Sakai, S., Yasuda, R., Sayo, T., Ishikawa, O. & Inoue, S. Hyaluronan Exists in the Normal Stratum Corneum. *J. Invest. Dermatol.* 114, 1184–1187 (2000).

[15] Verdier-Sévrain, S. & Bonté, F. Skin hydration: a review on its molecular mechanisms. *J. Cosmet. Dermatol.* 6, 75–82 (2007).

[16] Sougrat, R. et al., Functional Expression of AQP3 in Human Skin Epidermis and Reconstructed Epidermis. *J. Invest. Dermatol.* 118, 678–685 (2002).

[17] Fluhr, J. W. et al., Comparative study of five instruments measuring stratum corneum hydration (Corneometer CM 820 and CM 825, Skicon 200, Nova DPM 9003, DermaLab). Part I. In vitro. *Skin Res. Technol.* 5, 161–170 (1999).

[18] Tagami, H. et al., Water Sorption-desorption Test of the Skin in Vivo for Functional Assessment of the Stratum Corneum. *J. Invest. Dermatol.* 78, 425–428 (1982).

[19] Edwards, E. A. & Duntley, S. Q. The pigments and color of living human skin. *Am. J. Anat.* 65, 1–33 (1939).

[20] Kollias, N. & Stamatas, G. Optical Non-Invasive Approaches to Diagnosis of Skin Diseases. *J. Investig. Dermatol. Symp. Proc.* 7, 64–75 (2002).

[21] Reich, G. Near-infrared spectroscopy and imaging: Basic principles and pharmaceutical applications. *Adv. Drug Deliv. Rev.* 57, 1109–1143 (2005).

[22] Guillard, E. C., Tfayli, A., Laugel, C. & Baillet-Guffroy, A. Molecular interactions of penetration enhancers within ceramides organization: A FTIR approach. *Eur. J. Pharm. Sci.* 36, 192–199 (2009).

[23] Raman, C. V. & Krishnan, K. S. A New Type of Secondary Radiation. *Nature* 121, 501–502 (1928).

[24] Tfayli, A., Piot, O. & Manfait, M. Confocal Raman microspectroscopy on excised human skin: uncertainties in depth profiling and mathematical correction applied to dermatological drug permeation. *J. Biophotonics* 1, 140–153 (2008).

[25] Tfayli, A., Piot, O., Pitre, F. & Manfait, M. Follow-up of drug permeation through excised human skin with confocal Raman microspectroscopy. *Eur. Biophys. J.* 36, 1049–1058 (2007).

[26] Votteler, M., Carvajal Berrio, D. A., Pudlas, M., Walles, H. & Schenke-Layland, K. Non-contact, Label-free Monitoring of Cells and Extracellular Matrix using Raman Spectroscopy. *J. Vis. Exp. JoVE* (2012). doi:10.3791/3977

[27] Brancaleon, L., Lin, G. & Kollias, N. The In Vivo Fluorescence of Tryptophan Moieties in Human Skin Increases with UV Exposure and is a Marker for Epidermal Proliferation. *J. Invest. Dermatol.* 113, 977–982 (1999).

[28] Brancaleon, L. et al., In vivo Fluorescence Spectroscopy of Nonmelanoma Skin Cancer¶. *Photochem. Photobiol.* 73, 178–183 (2001).
[29] Doukas, A. G., Soukos, N. S., Babusis, S., Appa, Y. & Kollias, N. Fluorescence Excitation Spectroscopy for the Measurement of Epidermal Proliferation¶. *Photochem. Photobiol.* 74, 96–102 (2001).
[30] Gillies, R., Zonios, G., Anderson, R. R. & Kollias, N. Fluorescence Excitation Spectroscopy Provides Information About Human Skin In Vivo. *J. Invest. Dermatol.* 115, 704–707 (2000).
[31] González, S., Zonios, G., Nguyen, B. C., Gillies, R. & Kollias, N. Endogenous Skin Fluorescence is a Good Marker for Objective Evaluation of Comedolysis. *J. Invest. Dermatol.* 115, 100–105 (2000).
[32] Kollias, N. et al., Fluorescence photography in the evaluation of hyperpigmentation in photodamaged skin. *J. Am. Acad. Dermatol.* 36, 226–230 (1997).
[33] Kollias, N., Gillies, R., Moran, M., Kochevar, I. E. & Anderson, R. R. Endogenous Skin Fluorescence Includes Bands that may Serve as Quantitative Markers of Aging and Photoaging. *J. Invest. Dermatol.* 111, 776–780 (1998).
[34] Leffell, D., Stetz, M., Milstone, L. & Deckelbaum, L. In vivo fluorescence of human skin: A potential marker of photoaging. *Arch. Dermatol.* 124, 1514–1518 (1988).
[35] Lohmann, W. & Paul, E. In situ detection of melanomas by fluorescence measurements. *Naturwissenschaften* 75, 201–202 (1988).
[36] Lohmann, W. et al., Elastosis and cancer. *Z. Naturforschung C J. Biosci.* 49, 223–229 (1993).
[37] Richards-Kortum, R. & Sevick-Muraca, E. Quantitative Optical Spectroscopy for Tissue Diagnosis. *Annu. Rev. Phys. Chem.* 47, 555–606 (1996).
[38] Tian, W. D., Gillies, R., Brancaleon, L. & Kollias, N. Aging and Effects of Ultraviolet A Exposure may be Quantified by Fluorescence Excitation Spectroscopy In Vivo. *J. Invest. Dermatol.* 116, 840–845 (2001).
[39] Zeng, H., MacAulay, C., McLean, D. I., Palcic, B. & Lui, H. The Dynamics of Laser-Induced Changes in Human Skin Autofluorescence—Experimental Measurements and Theoretical Modeling. *Photochem. Photobiol.* 68, 227–236 (1998).
[40] Marchesini, R. et al., In vivo spectrophotometric evaluation of neoplastic and non-neoplastic skin pigmented lesions-I.Reflectance measurements. *Photochem. Photobiol.* 53, 77–84 (1991).

[41] Farkas, D. L. & Becker, D. Applications of Spectral Imaging: Detection and Analysis of Human Melanoma and Its Precursors. *Pigment Cell Res.* 14, 2–8 (2001).

[42] Draux, F. et al., Raman spectral imaging of single living cancer cells: a preliminary study. *Analyst* 134, 542–548 (2009).

[43] Rajadhyaksha, M., Grossman, M., Esterowitz, D., Webb, R. H. & Anderson, R. R. In Vivo Confocal Scanning Laser Microscopy of Human Skin: Melanin Provides Strong Contrast. *J. Invest. Dermatol.* 104, 946–952 (1995).

[44] Rajadhyaksha, M., González, S., Zavislan, J. M., Anderson, R. R. & Webb, R. H. In Vivo Confocal Scanning Laser Microscopy of Human Skin II: Advances in Instrumentation and Comparison With Histology1. *J. Invest. Dermatol.* 113, 293–303 (1999).

[45] Huzaira, M., Rius, F., Rajadhyaksha, M., Anderson, R. R. & González, S. Topographic Variations in Normal Skin, as Viewed by In Vivo Reflectance Confocal Microscopy. *J. Invest. Dermatol.* 116, 846–852 (2001).

[46] Gilchrest, B. a. & Yaar, M. Ageing and photoageing of the skin: observations at the cellular and molecular level. *Br. J. Dermatol.* 127, 25–30 (1992).

[47] Yaar, M. Molecular mechanisms of skin aging. *Adv. Dermatol.* 10, 63–75; discussion 76 (1994).

[48] Welzel, J., Reinhardt, C., Lankenau, E., Winter, C. & Wolff, H. h. Changes in function and morphology of normal human skin: evaluation using optical coherence tomography. *Br. J. Dermatol.* 150, 220–225 (2004).

[49] Pagnoni, A. et al., Optical coherence tomography in dermatology. *Skin Res. Technol.* 5, 83–87 (1999).

[50] Gambichler, T. et al., A Comparative Pilot Study on Ultraviolet-induced Skin Changes Assessed by Noninvasive Imaging Techniques in Vivo. *Photochem. Photobiol.* 82, 1103–1107 (2006).

[51] Sauermann, K. et al., Age related changes of human skin investigated with histometric measurements by confocal laser scanning microscopy in vivo. *Skin Res. Technol.* 8, 52–56 (2002).

[52] Corcuff, P., Bertrand, C. & Leveque, J. L. Morphometry of human epidermis in vivo by real-time confocal microscopy. *Arch. Dermatol. Res.* 285, 475–481 (1993).

[53] Gammal, S. E. et al., Sonography of the Skin at 100 MHz Enables In Vivo Visualization of Stratum Corneum and Viable Epidermis in Palmar Skin and Psoriatic Plaquesy1. *J. Invest. Dermatol.* 113, 821–829 (1999).

[54] Vogt, M., Knüttel, A., Hoffmann, K., Altmeyer, P. & Ermert, H. Comparison of High Frequency Ultrasound and Optical Coherence Tomography as Modalities for High Resolution and Non Invasive Skin Imaging. Vergleich von hochfrequentem Ultraschall und optischer Kohärenztomographie als Modalitäten für die hochauflösende und nichtinvasive Abbildung der Haut. *Biomed. Tech. Eng.* 48, 116–121 (2009).

[55] Gambichler, T. et al., Validation of optical coherence tomography in vivo using cryostat histology. *Phys. Med. Biol.* 52, N75 (2007).

[56] So, P. T. C., Dong, C. Y., Masters, B. R. & Berland, K. M. Two-Photon Excitation Fluorescence Microscopy. *Annu. Rev. Biomed. Eng.* 2, 399–429 (2000).

[57] Smeden, J. van et al., LC/MS analysis of stratum corneum lipids: ceramide profiling and discovery. *J. Lipid Res.* 52, 1211–1221 (2011).

[58] Merle, C., Laugel, C., Chaminade, P. & Baillet-Guffroy, A. Quantitative Study of the Stratum Corneum Lipid Classes by Normal Phase Liquid Chromatography: Comparison Between Two Universal Detectors. *J. Liq. Chromatogr. Relat. Technol.* 33, 629–644 (2010).

[59] Michael-Jubeli, R., Bleton, J. & Baillet-Guffroy, A. High-temperature gas chromatography-mass spectrometry for skin surface lipids profiling. *J. Lipid Res.* 52, 143–151 (2011).

[60] Masukawa, Y. et al., Characterization of overall ceramide species in human stratum corneum. *J. Lipid Res.* 49, 1466–1476 (2008).

[61] Masukawa, Y. et al., Comprehensive quantification of ceramide species in human stratum corneum. *J. Lipid Res.* 50, 1708–1719 (2009).

[62] Beauregard, S. & Gilchrest, B. A survey of skin problems and skin care regimens in the elderly. *Arch. Dermatol.* 123, 1638–1643 (1987).

[63] Dewberry, C. in *Diagnosis of Aging Skin Diseases* (ed. FAAIM, R. A. N. D., MPH) 99–105 (Springer London, 2008).

[64] Longo, C., Casari, A., Beretti, F., Cesinaro, A. M. & Pellacani, G. Skin aging: In vivo microscopic assessment of epidermal and dermal changes by means of confocal microscopy. *J. Am. Acad. Dermatol.* 68, e73–e82 (2013).

[65] Naylor, E. C., Watson, R. E. B. & Sherratt, M. J. Molecular aspects of skin ageing. *Maturitas* 69, 249–256 (2011).

[66] Farage, M. A. & Maibach, H. I. *The Vulva: Anatomy, Physiology, and Pathology*. (CRC Press, 2006).

[67] El-Domyati, M. et al., Intrinsic aging vs. photoaging: a comparative histopathological, immunohistochemical, and ultrastructural study of skin. *Exp. Dermatol.* 11, 398–405 (2002).

[68] Whitton, J. T. & Everall, J. d. The thickness of the epidermis. *Br. J. Dermatol.* 89, 467–476 (1973).

[69] Marks, R. Measurement of biological ageing in human epidermis. *Br. J. Dermatol.* 104, 627–633 (1981).

[70] Lock-Andersen, J. et al., Epidermal thickness, skin pigmentation and constitutive photosensitivity. *Photodermatol. Photoimmunol. Photomed.* 13, 153–158 (1997).

[71] Boireau-Adamezyk, E., Baillet-Guffroy, A. & Stamatas, G. N. Age-dependent changes in stratum corneum barrier function. *Skin Res. Technol.* n/a–n/a (2014). doi:10.1111/srt.12132

[72] Lavker, R. M. & Kligman, A. M. Chronic Heliodermatitis: A Morphologic Evaluation of Chronic Actinic Dermal Damage With Emphasis on the Role of Mast Cells. *J. Invest. Dermatol.* 90, 325–330 (1988).

[73] Lavker, R. M. Structural Alterations in Exposed and Unexposed Aged Skin. *J. Invest. Dermatol.* 73, 59–66 (1979).

[74] Branchet, M. C., Boisnic, S., Frances, C. & Robert, A. M. Skin Thickness Changes in Normal Aging Skin. *Gerontology* 36, 28–35 (1990).

[75] Harvell, J. D. & Maibach, H. I. Percutaneous absorption and inflammation in aged skin: A review. *J. Am. Acad. Dermatol.* 31, 1015–1021 (1994).

[76] Sans, M. & Moraga, A. Mathematical morphologic analysis of the aortic medial structure. Biomechanical implications. *Anal. Quant. Cytol. Histol. Int. Acad. Cytol. Am. Soc. Cytol.* 15, 93–100 (1993).

[77] Waller, J. M. & Maibach, H. I. Age and skin structure and function, a quantitative approach (I): blood flow, pH, thickness, and ultrasound echogenicity. *Skin Res. Technol.* 11, 221–235 (2005).

[78] Oriba, H. a., Bucks, D. a. w. & Maibach, H. i. Percutaneous absorption of hydrocortisone and testosterone on the vulva and forearm: effect of the menopause and site. *Br. J. Dermatol.* 134, 229–233 (1996).

[79] Robert, C., Blanc, M., Lesty, C., Dikstein, S. & Robert, L. Study of Skin Ageing as a Function of Social and Professional Conditions:

Modification of the Rheological Parameters Measured with a Noninvasive Method – Indentometry. *Gerontology* 34, 284–290 (1988).

[80] Ghadially, R., Brown, B. E., Sequeira-Martin, S. M., Feingold, K. R. & Elias, P. M. The aged epidermal permeability barrier. Structural, functional, and lipid biochemical abnormalities in humans and a senescent murine model. *J. Clin. Invest.* 95, 2281–2290 (1995).

[81] Roskos, K. V. & Guy, R. H. Assessment of Skin Barrier Function Using Transepidermal Water Loss: Effect of Age. *Pharm. Res.* 6, 949–953 (1989).

[82] Haratake, A., Uchida, Y., Mimura, K., Elias, P. M. & Holleran, W. M. Intrinsically Aged Epidermis Displays Diminished UVB-Induced Alterations in Barrier Function Associated with decreased Proliferation. *J. Invest. Dermatol.* 108, 319–323 (1997).

[83] Wilhelm KP, Cua AB & Maibach HI. Skin aging: Effect on transepidermal water loss, stratum corneum hydration, skin surface ph, and casual sebum content. *Arch. Dermatol.* 127, 1806–1809 (1991).

[84] Berardesca, E. & Maibach, H. I. Transepidermal water loss and skin surface hydration in the non invasive assessment of stratum corneum function. *Dermatosen Beruf Umw. Occup. Environ.* 38, 50–53 (1990).

[85] Cua, A. B., Wilhelm, K.-P. & Maibach, H. i. Frictional properties of human skin: relation to age, sex and anatomical region, stratum corneum hydration and transepidermal water loss. *Br. J. Dermatol.* 123, 473–479 (1990).

[86] Kobayashi, H. & Tagami, H. Distinct locational differences observable in biophysical functions of the facial skin: with special emphasis on the poor functional properties of the stratum corneum of the perioral region. *Int. J. Cosmet. Sci.* 26, 91–101 (2004).

[87] Stamatas, G. N. & Boireau-Adamezyk, E. Development of a Non-Invasive Optical Method for Assessment of Skin Barrier to External Penetration. in *Biomedical Optics and 3-D Imaging* JM3A.42 (Optical Society of America, 2012). doi:10.1364/BIOMED.2012.JM3A.42

[88] Cua, A. B., Wilhelm, K.-P. & Maibach, H. I. Skin Surface Lipid and Skin Friction: Relation to Age, Sex and Anatomical Region. *Skin Pharmacol. Physiol.* 8, 246–251 (1995).

[89] Schreiner, V. et al., Barrier Characteristics of Different Human Skin Types Investigated with X-Ray Diffraction, Lipid Analysis, and Electron Microscopy Imaging. *J. Invest. Dermatol.* 114, 654–660 (2000).

[90] Roskos, K., Guy, R. & Maibach, H. Percutaneous absorption in the aged. *Dermatol. Clin.* 4, 455–465 (1986).

[91] Rogers, J., Harding, C., Mayo, A., Banks, J. & Rawlings, A. Stratum corneum lipids: the effect of ageing and the seasons. *Arch. Dermatol. Res.* 288, 765–770 (1996).
[92] Saint Léger, D. et al., Age-associated changes in stratum corneum lipids and their relation to dryness. *Dermatologica* 177, 159–164 (1987).
[93] Denda, M. et al., Age- and sex-dependent change in stratum corneum sphingolipids. *Arch. Dermatol. Res.* 285, 415–417 (1993).
[94] Rabionet, M., Gorgas, K. & Sandhoff, R. Ceramide synthesis in the epidermis. *Biochim. Biophys. Acta BBA - Mol. Cell Biol. Lipids* 1841, 422–434 (2014).
[95] Grove, G. L. & Kligman, A. M. Age-associated Changes in Human Epidermal Cell Renewal. *J. Gerontol.* 38, 137–142 (1983).
[96] Roskos, K. V. The effect of skin aging on the percutaneous penetration of chemicals through human skin. (1989).
[97] Makrantonaki, E. & Zouboulis, C. C. Molecular Mechanisms of Skin Aging. *Ann. N. Y. Acad. Sci.* 1119, 40–50 (2007).
[98] Ghadially, R. et al., Decreased Epidermal Lipid Synthesis Accounts for Altered Barrier Function in Aged Mice. *J. Invest. Dermatol.* 106, 1064–1069 (1996).
[99] Man M, Feingold KR & Elias PM. EXogenous lipids influence permeability barrier recovery in acetone-treated murine skin. *Arch. Dermatol.* 129, 728–738 (1993).
[100] Potts, R. O. & Francoeur, M. L. The Influence of Stratum Corneum Morphology on Water Permeability. *J. Invest. Dermatol.* 96, 495–499 (1991).
[101] Denda, M., Koyama, J., Namba, R. & Horii, I. Stratum corneum lipid morphology and transepidermal water loss in normal skin and surfactant-induced scaly skin. *Arch. Dermatol. Res.* 286, 41–46 (1994).
[102] Elias, P. & Menon, G. Structural and lipid biochemical correlates of the epidermal permeability barrier. *Adv. Lipid Res.* 24, 1–26 (1990).
[103] Golden, G. M., Guzek, D. B., Kennedy, A. E., McKie, J. E. & Potts, R. O. Stratum corneum lipid phase transitions and water barrier properties. *Biochemistry (Mosc.)* 26, 2382–2388 (1987).
[104] Guillard, E., Tfayli, A., Manfait, M. & Baillet-Guffroy, A. Thermal dependence of Raman descriptors of ceramides. Part II: effect of chains lengths and head group structures. *Anal. Bioanal. Chem.* 399, 1201–1213 (2010).
[105] Lawson, E. E., Anigbogu, A. N. C., Williams, A. C., Barry, B. W. & Edwards, H. G. M. Thermally induced molecular disorder in human

stratum corneum lipids compared with a model phospholipid system; FT-Raman spectroscopy. *Spectrochim. Acta. A. Mol. Biomol. Spectrosc.* 54, 543–558 (1998).

[106] Tfayli, A., Guillard, E., Manfait, M. & Baillet-Guffroy, A. Thermal dependence of Raman descriptors of ceramides. Part I: effect of double bonds in hydrocarbon chains. *Anal. Bioanal. Chem.* 397, 1281–1296 (2010).

[107] Tfayli, A., Guillard, E., Manfait, M. & Baillet-Guffroy, A. Raman spectroscopy: feasibility of in vivo survey of stratum corneum lipids, effect of natural aging. *Eur. J. Dermatol. EJD* 22, 36–41 (2012).

[108] Le Fur, I. et al., Analysis of Circadian and Ultradian Rhythms of Skin Surface Properties of Face and Forearm of Healthy Women. *J. Invest. Dermatol.* 117, 718–724 (2001).

[109] Fenske, N. A. & Lober, C. W. Structural and functional changes of normal aging skin. *J. Am. Acad. Dermatol.* 15, 571–585 (1986).

[110] Henderson, C. a., Taylor, J. & Cunliffe, W. j. Sebum excretion rates in mothers and neonates. *Br. J. Dermatol.* 142, 110–111 (2000).

[111] Pochi, P. E., Strauss, J. S. & Downing, D. T. Age-related Changes in Sebaceous Gland Activity. *J. Invest. Dermatol.* 73, 108–111 (1979).

[112] Pochi, P. E. & Strauss, J. S. Endocrinologic Control to the Development and Activity of the Human Sebaceous Gland. *J. Invest. Dermatol.* 62, 191–201 (1974).

[113] Dieudonne, M. N., Pecquery, R., Leneveu, M. C. & Giudicelli, Y. Opposite Effects of Androgens and Estrogens on Adipogenesis in Rat Preadipocytes: Evidence for Sex and Site-Related Specificities and Possible Involvement of Insulin-Like Growth Factor 1 Receptor and Peroxisome Proliferator-Activated Receptorγ 2. *Endocrinology* 141, 649–656 (2000).

[114] Tavakkol, A., Varani, J., Elder, J. T. & Zouboulis, C. C. Maintenance of human skin in organ culture: role for insulin-like growth factor-1 receptor and epidermal growth factor receptor. *Arch. Dermatol. Res.* 291, 643–651 (1999).

[115] Plewig, G. & Kligman, A. M. Proliferative Activity of the Sebaceous Glands of the Aged. *J. Invest. Dermatol.* 70, 314–317 (1978).

[116] Zlotogorski, A. Distribution of skin surface pH on the forehead and cheek of adults. *Arch. Dermatol. Res.* 279, 398–401 (1987).

[117] Denda, M., Tomitaka, A., Akamatsu, H. & Matsunaga, K. Altered Distribution of Calcium in Facial Epidermis of Aged Adults. *J. Invest. Dermatol.* 121, 1557–1558 (2003).

[118] Reed, J., Elias, P. & Ghadially, R. Integrity and permeability barrier function of photoaged human epidermis. *Arch. Dermatol.* 133, 395–396 (1997).
[119] Eaglstein, W. Wound healing and aging. *Clin. Geriatr. Med.* 5, 183–188 (1989).
[120] Kligman, A. M. The treatment of photoaged human skin by topical tretinoin. *Drugs* 38, 1–8 (1989).
[121] Grove, G. Physiologic changes in older skin. *Clin. Geriatr. Med.* 5, 115–125 (1989).
[122] Eisner, P., Wilhelm, D. & Maibach, H. I. Frictional Properties of Human Forearm and Vulvar Skin: Influence of Age and Correlation with Transepidermal Water Loss and Capacitance. *Dermatology* 181, 88–91 (1990).
[123] Potts, R. O., Buras, E. M. & Chrisman, D. A. Changes with Age in the Moisture Content of Human Skin. *J. Invest. Dermatol.* 82, 97–100 (1984).
[124] Walrafen, G. E. in *The Physics and Physical Chemistry of Water* (ed. Franks, F.) 151–214 (Springer New York, 1972).
[125] Nielsen, O. F. The structure of liquid water. A low frequency (10–400 cm−1) Raman study. *Chem. Phys. Lett.* 60, 515–517 (1979).
[126] Nielsen, O. F. Chapter 2. Low-frequency spetroscopic studies of interactions in liquids. *Annu. Rep. Sect. C Phys. Chem.* 90, 3–44 (1993).
[127] Nielsen, O. F., Christensen, D. H., Trandum, C., Gniadecka, M. & Wulf, H. C. in *Spectroscopy of Biological Molecules: Modern Trends* (eds. Carmona, P., Navarro, R. & Hernanz, A.) 593–594 (Springer Netherlands, 1997).
[128] Maeda, Y. & Kitano, H. The structure of water in polymer systems as revealed by Raman spectroscopy. *Spectrochim. Acta. A. Mol. Biomol. Spectrosc.* 51, 2433–2446 (1995).
[129] Gniadecka, M. et al., Water and Protein Structure in Photoaged and Chronically Aged Skin. *J. Invest. Dermatol.* 111, 1129–1132 (1998).
[130] Gniadecka, M., Nielsen, O. F., Christensen, D. H. & Wulf, H. C. Structure of Water, Proteins, and Lipids in Intact Human Skin, Hair, and Nail. *J. Invest. Dermatol.* 110, 393–398 (1998).
[131] Cavatorta, F., Fontana, M. P. & Vecli, A. Raman spectroscopy of protein–water interactions in aqueous solutions. *J. Chem. Phys.* 65, 3635–3640 (1976).

[132] Vyumvuhore, R. et al., Effects of atmospheric relative humidity on Stratum Corneum structure at the molecular level: ex vivo Raman spectroscopy analysis. *Analyst* 138, 4103–4111 (2013).

[133] Boireau-Adamezyk, E., Baillet-Guffroy, A. & Stamatas, G. N. Mobility of Water Molecules in the Stratum Corneum: Effects of Age and Chronic Exposure to the Environment. *J. Invest. Dermatol.* 134, 2046–2049 (2014).

[134] Bulgin, J. J. & Vinson, L. J. The use of differential thermal analysis to study the bound water in stratum corneum membranes. *Biochim. Biophys. Acta BBA - Gen. Subj.* 136, 551–560 (1967).

[135] Egawa, M. & Tagami, H. Comparison of the depth profiles of water and water-binding substances in the stratum corneum determined in vivo by Raman spectroscopy between the cheek and volar forearm skin: effects of age, seasonal changes and artificial forced hydration. *Br. J. Dermatol.* 158, 251–260 (2008).

[136] Sauermann, K., Jaspers, S., Koop, U. & Wenck, H. Topically applied vitamin C increases the density of dermal papillae in aged human skin. *BMC Dermatol.* 4, 13 (2004).

[137] McCullough, J. L. & Kristen M., K. Prevention and Treatment of Skin Aging. *Ann. N. Y. Acad. Sci.* 1067, 323–331 (2006).

[138] Marks, R., Lawson, A. & Nicholls, S. in *Stratum Corneum* (eds. Marks, P. R. & Plewig, P. D. G.) 175–180 (Springer Berlin Heidelberg, 1983).

[139] Vyumvuhore, R. et al., The relationship between water loss, mechanical stress, and molecular structure of human stratum corneum ex vivo: Relationship between SC water loss, mechanical stress, and molecular structure. *J. Biophotonics* n/a–n/a (2014). doi:10.1002/jbio.201300169

[140] Baker, H. & Blair, C. P. Cell Replacement in the Human Stratum Corneum in Old Age. *Br. J. Dermatol.* 80, 367–372 (1968).

[141] Suter-Widmer, J. & Elsner. The Irritant Contact Dermatits Syndrome. *Boca Raton: CRC Press* (1996).

[142] Wu, J. Q. & Kilpatrick-Liverman, L. Characterizing the composition of underarm and forearm skin using confocal raman spectrscopy. *Int. J. Cosmet. Sci.* 33, 257–262 (2011).

[143] Oh, J.-H. et al., Intrinsic aging- and photoaging-dependent level changes of glycosaminoglycans and their correlation with water content in human skin. *J. Dermatol. Sci.* 62, 192–201 (2011).

[144] Tammi, R., Ripellino, J. A., Margolis, R. U. & Tammi, M. Localization of Epidermal Hyaluronic Acid Using the Hyaluronate Binding Region of

Cartilage Proteoglycan as a Specific Probe. *J. Invest. Dermatol.* 90, 412–414 (1988).

[145] Kohen, R. & Gati, I. Skin low molecular weight antioxidants and their role in aging and in oxidative stress. *Toxicology* 148, 149–157 (2000).

[146] Lopez-Torres, M., Shindo, Y. & Packer, L. Effect of Age on Antioxidants and Molecular Markers of Oxidative Damage in Murine Epidermis and Dermis. *J. Invest. Dermatol.* 102, 476–480 (1994).

[147] Wei, Y., Lu, C., Wei, C., Ma, Y. & Lee, H. Oxidative stress in human aging and mitochondrial disease-consequences of defective mitochondrial respiration and impaired antioxidant enzyme system. *Chin. J. Physiol.* 44, 1–11 (2001).

[148] Lemire, J. M. Immunomodulatory actions of 1,25-Dihydroxyvitamin D3. *J. Steroid Biochem. Mol. Biol.* 53, 599–602 (1995).

[149] D'Ambrosio, D. et al., Inhibition of IL-12 production by 1,25-dihydroxyvitamin D3. Involvement of NF-kappaB downregulation in transcriptional repression of the p40 gene. *J. Clin. Invest.* 101, 252–262 (1998).

[150] Cerimele, D., Celleno, L. & Serri, F. Physiological changes in ageing skin. *Br. J. Dermatol.* 122, 13–20 (1990).

[151] Sunderkötter, C., Kalden, H. & Luger, T. AGing and the skin immune system. *Arch. Dermatol.* 133, 1256–1262 (1997).

[152] Ye, J. et al., Alterations in cytokine regulation in aged epidermis: implications for permeability barrier homeostasis and inflammation. *Exp. Dermatol.* 11, 209–216 (2002).

[153] Reinboth, B., Hanssen, E., Cleary, E. G. & Gibson, M. A. Molecular Interactions of Biglycan and Decorin with Elastic Fiber Components Biglycan forms a ternary complex with tropoelastin and microfibril-associated glycoprotein 1. *J. Biol. Chem.* 277, 3950–3957 (2002).

[154] Elias, P. M. & Ghadially, R. The Aged Epidermal Permeability Barrier. *Clin. Geriatr. Med.* 18, 103–120 (2002).

[155] Kligman, L. & Kligman, A. The nature of photoaging: its prevention and repair. *Photodermatol.* 3, 215–227 (1986).

[156] Gilchrest, B. a. A review of skin ageing and its medical therapy. *Br. J. Dermatol.* 135, 867–875 (1996).

[157] Benedetto, A. V. The environment and skin aging. *Clin. Dermatol.* 16, 129–139 (1998).

[158] Kang, S., Fisher, G. & Voorhees, J. Photoaging and topical tretinoin: Therapy, pathogenesis, and prevention. *Arch. Dermatol.* 133, 1280–1284 (1997).

[159] Südel, K. M. et al., Novel Aspects of Intrinsic and Extrinsic Aging of Human Skin: Beneficial Effects of Soy Extract¶. *Photochem. Photobiol.* 81, 581–587 (2005).

[160] Robinson, M. K. Population differences in skin structure and physiology and the susceptibility to irritant and allergic contact dermatitis: implications for skin safety testing and risk assessment. *Contact Dermatitis* 41, 65–79 (1999).

[161] Glogau, R. G. Physiologic and structural changes associated with aging skin. *Dermatol. Clin.* 15, 555–559 (1997).

[162] Bergfeld, W. The aging skin. *Int. J. Fertil. Womens Med.* 42, 57–66 (1996).

[163] Gniadecka, M., Wulf, H., Mortensen, N. & Poulsen, T. Photoprotection in vitiligo and normal skin. A quantitative assessment of the role of stratum corneum, viable epidermis and pigmentation. *Acta Derm. Venereol.* 76, 429–432 (1996).

[164] Kohno, Y. et al., Kinetic study of quenching reaction of singlet oxygen and scavenging reaction of free radical by squalene in n-butanol. *Biochim. Biophys. Acta BBA - Lipids Lipid Metab.* 1256, 52–56 (1995).

[165] Pelle, E., Muizzuddin, N., Mammone, T., Marenus, K. & Maes, D. Protection against endogenous and UVB-induced oxidative damage in stratum corneum lipids by an antioxidant-containing cosmetic formulation. *Photodermatol. Photoimmunol. Photomed.* 15, 115–119 (1999).

[166] Saint-Leger, D., Bague, A., Lefebvre, E., Cohen, E. & Chivot, M. A possible role for squalene in the pathogenesis of acne. II. In vivo study of squalene oxides in skin surface and intra-comedonal lipids of acne patients. *Br. J. Dermatol.* 114, 543–552 (1986).

[167] Harwood, C. A. et al., An Association Between Sebaceous Carcinoma and Microsatellite Instability in Immunosuppressed Organ Transplant Recipients. *J. Invest. Dermatol.* 116, 246–253 (2001).

[168] MacLaughlin, J. & Holick, M. F. Aging decreases the capacity of human skin to produce vitamin D3. *J. Clin. Invest.* 76, 1536–1538 (1985).

[169] Gloth, F. et al., VItamin d deficiency in homebound elderly persons. *JAMA* 274, 1683–1686 (1995).

[170] Sander, C. S. et al., Photoaging is Associated with Protein Oxidation in Human Skin In Vivo. *J. Invest. Dermatol.* 118, 618–625 (2002).

[171] Thiele, J. J., Traber, M. G. & Packer, L. Depletion of Human Stratum Corneum Vitamin E: An Early and Sensitive In Vivo Marker of UV Induced Photo-Oxidation. *J. Invest. Dermatol.* 110, 756–761 (1998).

[172] Hellemans, L., Corstjens, H., Neven, A., Declercq, L. & Maes, D. Antioxidant Enzyme Activity in Human Stratum Corneum Shows Seasonal Variation with an Age-Dependent Recovery. *J. Invest. Dermatol.* 120, 434–439 (2003).
[173] Kondo, S. The Roles of Keratinocyte-Derived Cytokines in the Epidermis and Their Possible Responses to UVA-Irradiation. *J. Investig. Dermatol. Symp. Proc.* 4, 177–183 (1999).
[174] Kondo, S. The roles of cytokines in photoaging. *J. Dermatol. Sci.* 23, Supplement 1, S30–S36 (2000).
[175] Jenkins, G. Molecular mechanisms of skin ageing. *Mech. Ageing Dev.* 123, 801–810 (2002).
[176] Model, D. Smoker's face: an underrated clinical sign? *Br. Med. J. Clin. Res. Ed* 291, 1760–1762 (1985).
[177] Placzek, M., Kerkmann, U., Bell, S., Koepke, P. & Przybilla, B. Tobacco smoke is phototoxic. *Br. J. Dermatol.* 150, 991–993 (2004).
[178] Ernster, V. L. et al., Facial wrinkling in men and women, by smoking status. *Am. J. Public Health* 85, 78–82 (1995).

In: Skin Aging and Photoaging
Editor: Emanuel Graham

ISBN: 978-1-63482-907-6

Chapter 6

Polyphenolic Nanobiomaterials As Emerging Therapies for Combating Physiology and Clinical Aspects of Photoaging and Photocarcinogenesis

Neena Philips*[*]*, PhD, Jovinna Chalensouk-Khaosaat, Avani Devmurrai and Hardika Patel
Fairleigh Dickinson University, Teaneck, NJ, US

Abstract

The physiology of skin photoaging and photocarcinogenesis is due to oxidative stress and inflammation, as well as direct damage to biomolecules, due to exposure to solar ultraviolet (UV) radiation. Additional factors include environmental pollutants, allergens such as disperse blue dyes, cigarette smoking and intrinsic aging. The clinical characteristics of photoaging and photocarcinogenesis are primarily due to the breakdown of the extracellular matrix (ECM), composed of collagen and elastin, by the stimulation of proteolytic enzymes, elastases

[*] Corresponding author: Neena Philips, Ph.D., Professor of Biology, Fairleigh Dickinson University, Teaneck, NJ 07666, nphilips@fdu.edu, neenaphilips@optonline.net, http://alpha.fdu.edu/~nphilips/

and matrixmetalloproteinases (MMP). Cellular oxidative stress, from reactive oxygen species, and inflammatory cytokines, including tumor necrosis factor-α (TNF- α), interleukin-1 (IL-1) and interleukin-6 (IL-6), alter signal transduction pathways such as the mitogen- activated protein kinase (MAPK), the JAK/STAT (Signal Transduction and Activation of Transcription), and the nuclear factor-kappa beta (NF-κB)/p65 that mediate the alterations in the ECM. A photoprotective strategy to counteract the mechanisms that lead to photoaging and photocarcinogenesis is prevention or treatment with polyphenolic phytochemicals, including those from *H. humulus* (xanthohumol) or *P. leucotomos,* which function as antioxidant and anti-inflammatory actives. A limitation of the photoprotective strategy with polyphenols is their topical or oral bioavailability (through absorption or assimilation) for efficacy. The emerging therapies are the delivery of polyphenols in biologically compatible nanomaterials, such as chitosan, polymeric nanoparticles/ micelles, nanoconjugates, liposomes, graphene, and phage systems. Polyphenols encapsulated in nanobiomaterial provide stronger antioxidant and anti-inflammatory activities, and thereby effectiveness to combat the physiology and clinical manifestations of photoaging and photocarcinogenesis.

Keywords: Collage, elastin, matrixmetalloproteinases, aging, cancer, polyphenols

Introduction

The physiology of photoaging and photocarcinogenesis is compromise to the integrity of the extracellular matrix (ECM). The ECM is composed of structural collagen and elastin fibers, which are degraded by matrixmetalloproteinases (MMP). The deterioration and remodeling of the ECM manifests as wrinkles, brown spots and skin atrophy in aging; and as angiogenesis for metastasis in cancer. The predominant mediators are oxidative stress and inflammation, which alter the expression of growth factors and cytokines that activate cellular signal transduction pathways to alter gene expression and thereby the ECM. Polyphenols are effective antioxidants and anti-inflammatory agents, with emerging therapies for enhanced effectiveness through encapsulation in nanobiomaterials.

1. Extracellular Matrix (ECM)

The collagen and elastin fibers provide the skin with strength, elasticity and resilience, and maintain the structural integrity of the skin. Skin aging and cancer are primarily from the deterioration of the ECM network due to reduced expression of collagen and elastin genes, and increased expression and activity of the MMPs.

I.1. Collagen

The collagen fibers are the predominant ECM structural proteins, in the interstitium as well as the basement membrane. There are 29 types of collagen, whose properties and classification are based on the lengths of the triple helical segments and amino acid composition or modifications. They are classified as fibrillar collagens, fibril associated collagens, sheet forming anchoring collagens, transmembrane collagens, and host defense collagens (Lodish et al., 2008). The predominant interstitial collagens in the skin are the fibrillar type I collagen (90%), and then types III and V collagens, and these are synthesized by dermal fibroblasts (Callaghan 2008, Philips et al., 2009b, Philips et al., 2010b).

I.2. Elastin

Elastin provides skin with elasticity and resilience. It is composed of elastin (90%) and fibrillin (Mecham et al., 1994). Fibrillin forms a microfibrillar scaffold for tropoelastin, and is crosslinked to it by lysyl oxidase and transglutaminase (Keeley et al., 2002, Kielty et al., 2002, Rock et al., 2004). Elastin is rich in proline, valine, lysine, alanine, glycine, leucine and isoleucine, while fibrillin is rich in cysteine that enables it to form a large number of disulphide bonds for its structure (Mecham et al., 1994, Kielty et al., 2002). The predominant microfibrils are fibrillin-1 and fibrillin-2, and are known to bind calcium and sequester growth factors such as transforming growth factor- β (TGF-β), which is key to regulating the expression of ECM proteins (Bax et al., 2003, Hubmacher et al., 2006, Kielty et al., 2002, Kinsey et al., 2008, Robert et al., 2002, Philips et al., 2009a, Philips et al., 2009b).

I.3. Matrixmetalloproteinases/Elastases

Collagen and elastin are degraded by matrixmetalloproteinases (MMP) and elastase. These proteases are produced by epidermal keratinocytes, dermal fibroblasts, and neutrophils in response to oxidative stress and inflammation (Brennan et al., 2003, Cho et al., 2007, Doyle et al., 1997, Jimenez et al., 2006, Khorramizadeh et al., 1999, Labat-Robert et al., 2000, Lee et al., 2008, Philips et al., 2004a, Philips et al., 2007, Philips et al., 2009a).

The MMPs are classified based on their substrate specificity or on their promoter sequences. MMPs are classified into groups based on their substrate specificity for fibrillar collagen, basement membrane proteins, pro-MMPs or elastin as collagenases, including MMP-1; gelatinases, including MMP-2 and 9; stromelysines, including MMP-3, and 10; the membrane-type MMPs; and other MMPs, including MMP-12 (Bode et al., 1993, Gomis-Rüth et al., 1996, Herouy et al., 2001, Nagase et al., 1999, Van Wart et al., 1990). The elastin fibers are predominantly degraded by elastases (Chakraborti et al., 2003, Kielty et al., 1994, Tsuji, 2001).

The MMPs are classified into groups based on the presence of TATA box and activator protein -1 (AP-1) transcription factor sequences as group I MMPs, including MMP-1, 3, 7, 9, 10, 12, 13, 19 and 26, which contain TATA box and AP-1 site; group II MMPs, including MMP-8, 11 and 21, which do not have the AP-1 site; and group III, including MMP-2, 14 and 28, which do not have the TATA box and AP-1 site (Yan et al., 2007). The MMPs are secreted as pro-MMPs, containing propeptide, catalytic, and C-terminal domains, and the proteolysis of the propeptide is essential for activity of MMPs (Bode et al., 1993, Gomis-Rüth et al., 1996, Herouy et al., 2001, Van Wart et al., 1990).

The MMPs are inhibited by the tissue inhibitors of MMPs (TIMP1, 2, 3 and 4) (Herouy et al., 2001, Verstappen et al., 2006).

Intrinsic aging, oxidative stress, inflammation, and ultraviolet (UV) radiation increase the expression and activities of MMPs and elastases and thereby facilitate aging and cancer (Fisher et al, 1996, Millis et al., 1992, Philips et al., 2007a, Philips et al., 2009a, Philips et al., 2009c, Philips et al., 2010a, Philips et al., 2010b).

2. Oxidative Stress and Inflammation

2.1. Oxidative Stress

Oxidative stress is a major cause of photoaging and cancer. Oxidative stress is due to the increased reactive oxygen species (ROS) from intrinsic aging, and exposure to environmental pollutants, allergens, cigarette smoke, and ultraviolet (UV) radiation. UV radiation is the predominant cause of increased ROS in photoaging and photocarcinogenesis. The solar UVA (320-400nm) radiation penetrates into the dermis; and although the UVB radiation (290-320 nm) penetrates only up to the dermis it has indirect effects on the dermal ECM (Krutmann, 2001, Nichols et al., 2010, Walscheck, 2001).

The ROS, including superoxide, hydroxyl radicals, hydrogen peroxide, and singlet oxygen, cause direct harm to biomolecules: to DNA to generate 8-oxo-7, 8-dihydro-2'-deoxyguanosine (8-oxo-dG), and pyrimidine dimmers, to proteins to form carbonyl amino acid derivatives, and to lipids to generate of lipid peroxides and lipid inflammatory mediators (Briganti et al., 2003, Callaghan et al., 2008, Melnikova et al., 2005, Nichols et al., 2010, Surjana et al., 2010). The ROS directly oxidize and glycate the ECM proteins, to compromise structure (Bailey et al., 2001, O'Rourke et al., 2007, Robert et al., 2008, Sims et al, 1996, Yaar et al., 2007).

2.2. Inflammation

Intrinsic factors and UV radiation, through ROS and other mechanisms, induce inflammatory cytokines [interleukin-1 (IL-1), interleukin-6 (IL-6), and tumor necrosis factor-α (TNF- α)] and growth factors [vascular endothelial growth factor (VEGF and TGF-β]. The inflammatory cytokines increase the expression of MMPs and VEGF, for ECM remodeling. VEGF is key to the formation of blood vessels; the leakage from which forms the dark spots in aging, and facilitates tumor metastasis (Ali et al., 2011, Sandler et al., 2012, Ushio-Fukai, 2006, Ushio-Fukai and Nakamura, 2008, Yang et al., 2012). VEGF antibodies or peptides inhibit angiogenesis, and cancer metastasis (Kargi et al., 2012, Karroum et al., 2012, Morera et al., 2010, Sandler et al., 2012, Wang et al., 2010). TGF-β stimulates the expression of MMPs in epithelial cells, and increases expression of VEGF that collectively facilitate carcinogenesis (Fuxe et al., 2012, Juárez et al., 2011, Merryman et al., 1998, Perrot et al., 2012, Philips et al., 2003, Philips et al., 2007).

3. Signal Transduction Pathways

Oxidative stress and inflammation cause the activation of the vascular endothelium to express cell adhesion molecules and secrete chemokines that activate leukocytes to adhere to the endothelium, through their activated integrin's, and enter the skin tissue (Kindt et al., 2007, Lodish et al., 2008). The activated leukocytes release the inflammatory cytokines. The activation of the vascular endothelium also activates the inflammatory plasma mediators, including plasminogen activator that facilitates proteolysis, and the lipid inflammatory mediators, including prostaglandins, thromboxane, and leukotrienes (Kindt et al., 2007). The oxidative stress and inflammatory mediators induce the release and activation of elastases and collagenases that degrade the ECM, and increase vascular permeability and dilation (Kindt et al., 2007). The tissue inflammation can also elicit a systemic response as manifested by increased levels of cortisone, C-reactive protein, and leukocytosis (increased white blood cells production) (Kindt et al., 2007).

The oxidative stress and inflammatory mediators, such as IL-1, IL-6, TNF- α, and VEGF, activate the mitogen activated protein kinase (MAPK), the Akt/Protein kinase B (PKB), and JAK/STAT (Signal Transduction and Activation of Transcription) by binding to tyrosine receptor kinases or cytokine receptors; whereas the oxidative stress and inflammation directly activates the NF-kB pathway (Callaghan et al., 2008, Kindt et al.,2007, Lodish et al., 2008, Meeran et al., 2008, Nichols et al., 2010). The activation of these pathways results in increased expression of MMPs and reduced cell apoptosis, for cancer progression.

3.1. MAPK Pathway

The MAPK pathway is activated through the activation of ras, by adapter proteins in response to the activation of receptor tyrosine kinases or cytokine receptors by oxidative stress and inflammatory mediators, that activates the extracellular signal-regulated kinase 1/2 (ERK1/2), c-Jun-N-terminal-kinase, and p38 proteins (Lodish et al., 2008). These in turn activate several transcription factors to regulate expression of genes (Lodish et al., 2008). A key transcription factor induced by the MAPK pathway is activator protein -1 (AP-1), which inhibits the transcription of type I collagen gene and stimulates the transcription of MMPs that degrade collagen (Callaghan et al., 2008, Fisher et al., 1996).

3.2. PKB Pathway

The PKB or Akt, a serine threonine kinase, is activated through the activation of PI-3 kinase by activated receptor tyrosine kinases or cytokine receptors (Lodish et al., 2008). The PKB regulates transcription of genes; and phosphorylates and inactivates pro-apoptotic proteins BAD and FOXO 3A (Lodish et al., 2008, Maiese et al., 2009). The inactivation of BAD, by protein 14-3-3, in turn causes the anti-apoptotic Bcl2/Bcl-xl to inactivate BAX (the mitochondrial membrane ion channel protein), and prevent the release of cytochrome C into the cytoplasm for the stimulation of the caspase cascade for apoptosis (Ahn et al., 2003, Lodish et al., 2008, Maiese et al., 2009).

3.3. STAT Pathway

The STAT transcription factor is activated by JAK kinase following activation of cytokine receptors, and it directly regulates the expression of genes (Lodish et al., 2008).

In addition, the pathway inhibits apoptosis and allows for cell proliferation by activating Bcl-x_L (Lodish et al., 2008).

3.4. NF-kB Pathway

The NF-kB pathway is activated through the binding of inflammatory cytokines to NF-kB receptors and the activation of cytoplasmic I-kB kinase, which causes the degradation of the inhibitor of NF-kB transcription factor and the translocation of NF-kB to the nucleus for the regulation of gene expression (Lodish et al., 2008).

Some of the regulated genes include the inflammatory cytokines, chemokines, inducible nitric oxide synthase, cyclooxygenase, and anti-apoptotic proteins (Kindt et al., 2007, Lodish et al., 2008, Meeran et al., 2008).

4. Polyphenols, Nanobiomaterials, and Polyphenolic Nanobiomaterials

4.1. Polyphenols

The increased ROS, in photoaging and photocarcinogenesis, cannot be counteracted solely by cellular antioxidants, including enzymes such as catalase and glutathione peroxidase, and small molecules such as glutathione, ascorbate, tocopherol, and carotene (Callaghan et al., 2008). Polyphenols have been identified as the major exogenous antioxidants to balance the increased ROS in photoaging and photocarcinogenesis. Phenolic compounds have an aromatic ring with one (monophenols) or more hydroxyl groups (polyphenols). They have ROS scavenging activity because of the hydroxyl groups. The diverse polyphenols inhibit the signal transduction pathways induced by oxidative and inflammatory factors and thereby counteract photoaging and photocarcinogenesis (Philips et al., 2013). The diverse polyphenols and their natural sources include xanthohumol from HOP plant (*H. lupulus)*, anthocyanin from grapes, catechins from tea leaves, isoflavones from soy, lignans from flax seeds, proanthocyanidins from red wine, procyanidins from apple, stilbenes from resveratrol, and tannins from nuts (Nichols et al., 2010; Philips et al., 2013). The polyphenols that have been extensively studied in my laboratory are xanthohumol, and those from *P. leucotomos.*

Xanthohumol is the major prenylated flavonoid isolated from the hop plant Humulus lupulus L. (Cannabinaceae) (Hops). From among the Hops components, xanthohumol is the most potent anti-cancer, anti-inflammatory and anti-oxidant compound. Xanthohumol is effective in preventing the initiation (chemopreventive) and progression of cancer (anti-carcinogenic). It's chemopreventive property is primarily from its anti-genotoxic mechanisms, inhibition of cytochrome P450 enzymes for activation of xenobiotics, stimulation of detoxification enzymes, and the activation of antioxidant response element (ARE) in genes (Luo et.al., 2007). Xanthohumol inhibits cancer progression by inhibiting cell proliferation as well as inducing apoptosis, upregulating cell adhesion molecules for anti-invasiveness, inhibiting DNA replication, and inhibiting drug efflux transporters (Delmulle et al., 2006, Lust et.al., 2005, Monteiro et al., 2007, Vanhoeke et al., 2005, Yang et al., 2007). The anti-inflammatory effects of xanthohumol include inhibition of cyclooxygenases and prostaglandins (Lemay et al., 2004). A major mechanism of xanthohumol effect is via the inhibition of NF-kB transcription factor (Colte et al., 2007). Xanthohumol stimulates the fibrillar collagens, elastin, and fibrillin in dermal fibroblasts (Philips et al., 2010b).

P. leucotomos is a fern, the extract of which is rich in polyphenols. It is marketed in topical and oral forms for photoprotection. It is rich in polyphenols that confers antioxidant and anti-inflammatory properties (Gonzalez et al., 1997, Gonzalez et al., 2000, Jańczyk et al., 2007, Philips et al., 1993, Philips et al., 2009). The stimulation of MMPs by cytotoxic ascorbate concentration is counteracted by *P. leucotomos* (Philips et al., 2009). *P. leucotomos* inhibits lipid peroxidation, and expression of MMPs, and stimulates the expression of fibrillar collagens, elastin, and TIMPs in fibroblasts or melanoma cells (Philips el al., 2003, Philips et al., 2009a).

4.2. Nanobiomaterials

The effectiveness of polyphenols is limited because of its low solubility or bioavailability topically and systemically. Nanobiomaterials improve delivery of actives as well as allow for targeted delivery, which is especially beneficial in treatment of cancer or for systemic administration of actives. The accumulation of actives in cancer tissue is by passive means of enhanced permeability and retention (EPR) effect, or from targeted delivery through the fusion of actives with antibodies or peptides (Jin et al., 2014). The ideal characteristics of nanobiomaterials include increased targeted bioavailability, stability and sustained release of actives, and the biodegradation and compatibility of the nanobiomaterials (Jin et al., 2014).

4.3. Polyphenolic Nanobiomaterials

The focus in the prevention of photoaging and photocarcinogenesis has been in the use of sunscreens, titanium dioxide (TiO_2), zinc oxide, and avobenzone, with micronized/nano TiO_2 providing the greatest safety and efficacy (Goodner et al., 2008). The focus is changing to bionanomaterials for the delivery of polyphenols; which can provide greater effectiveness of the polyphenol, from improved delivery into cells, and in addition biodegrade and thereby be less toxic to the cells and the environment (Berg et al., 2012, Ratner et al., 2004, Rosen et al., 2012). The nanobiomaterials that have been investigated for the effective delivery and effectiveness of polyphenols include chitosan, polymeric nanoparticles or micelles, nanoconjugates, liposomes, and carbon based nanoplatforms. An upcoming nanobiomaterial for investigation as polyphenolic nanobiomaterials, for delivery, can be the phage system.

A biomaterial used extensively in nanobiotechnology is ***chitosan/chitin.*** The properties of chitosan include biodegradability and compatibility, and in addition intrinsic beneficial effects on the ECM (Qin et al., 2010). Green tea polyphenols chitosan complex shows effective controlled release of its antioxidant property, through the inhibition of oxidative alteration of biomolecules, and the increased expression of transglutaminase genes for epithelial regeneration (Qin et al., 2010; Qin et al., 2013). Chitin Nanofibril-Hyaluronan (CN-HA) nanoparticles formulations are safe and effective for the delivery of actives (Liang XJ ., 2013, Morganti et al., 2013). The skin surface has a net negative charge, and the positive charge of the CN-HA increases delivery of the active to the interior of skin cells (Morganti et al., 2013, Morganti et al., 2012, Morganti P., 2009, Morganti P., 2010, Shin et al., 2010). An added advantage of CN-HA is skin hydration, an intrinsic property of HA. Red grape extract chitosan derivatives have improved intestinal absorption and effectiveness for endothelial health (Felice et al., 2012). The red grape extract chitosan HA derivative offers greater resistance to oxidation of endothelial progenitor cells (Felice et al., 2013). The prevalent polymeric nanobiomaterials are ***poly (lactide-co-glycolide) acid (PLGA),*** most widely used, and poly (ehylene glycol) (PEG) that was initially used to increase stability and thereby half-life of actives in blood (Jin et al., 2014). PLGA is biodegradable and biocompatible, and allows for controlled and targeted delivery of actives (Srivastava et al., 2013). Green tea polyphenols in PLGA nanoparticles show greater entrapment efficacy and prevention of chemical induced DNA damage and carcinogenesis through the induction of DNA repair genes and the inhibition of inflammatory mediators (Srivastava et al., 2013).

Nanoconjugates are mostly synthesized by conjugating functional groups or targets to polymers, for the purpose of targeted delivery of actives (Jin et al., 2014). The two prevalent conjugates are folate to target tumor cells, which have increased number of folate receptors, and albumin, which is small and has less cytotoxicity (Jin et al., 2014). Tannic acid cotton conjugate inhibits collagenase and inflammation (Perelshtein et al., 2014).

The ***liposomes*** provide a phospholipid bilayer, which allows hydrophilic actives to be carried in the hydrophilic interior and hydrophobic actives to be carried at its hydrophobic surface (Jin et al., 2014). Liposomes are used for passive or active targeting of actives, and are biocompatible and biodegradable (Jin et al., 2014). The hyperthermic property of tumor is used in the targeted delivery of actives by liposomes for cancer therapy (Jin et al., 2014). Tea polyphenol nanoliposome show sustained release of polyphenols, and antioxidant activity, as well as antibacterial activity (Zou et al., 2014).

Carbon based nanomaterial, which includes ***graphene,*** are multifunction and more conducive to engineering (Jin et al., 2014). Graphene is two dimensional, hydrophilic, used as reduced graphene oxide for targeted delivery of actives, as well as hybrids with other nanobiomaterials (Jun et al., 2014). Green tea polyphenols graphene nanosheets specifically target cancer cells for enhanced photo-destruction (Abdolahad et al., 2013). An upcoming nanobiomaterial for the delivery of actives is ***phage system.*** Bacteriophages have a simple structure, most consisting of a protein coat encompassing genetic information as DNA or RNA and essential enzyme. Bacteriophages have been used in recombinant DNA technology for cloning genes (Lodish et al., 2008). They can attach to hosts and inject their genetic material into the hosts, for replication and gene expression and thereby propagation. They can be assembled in-vitro. Hence bacteriophages provide an effective means of targeted delivery of actives through the engineering of targets to the coat proteins of bacteriophages, which can encompass the active, for delivery (Liu et al., 2012, Jin et al., 2014). The nanobiomaterials, chitosan, polymeric nanoparticles/ micelles, nanoconjugates, liposomes, graphene, and viral phages, may be suitable for use for improving the delivery of polyphenols, including xanthohumol and *P. leucotomos* extract, to combat the physiology and thereby clinical manifestations of photoaging and photocarcinogenesis.

Conclusion

The physiology of photoaging and photocarcinogenesis is primarily from the degradation of the structural collagen and elastin fibers of the ECM by MMPs due to increased cellular oxidative stress and inflammation from intrinsic factors and exposure to UV radiation, which activate MAPK, Akt/Protein kinase B (PKB), JAK/STAT, and NF-kB/p65, pathways to alter the expression of the ECM genes (Figure 1). The clinical manifestations include wrinkles, dark spots, and impaired wound healing with aging; and angiogenesis and cell proliferation that facilitate carcinogenesis (Figure 1). Polyphenols, including xanthohumol, *P. Leucotomos* extract, catechins/tannin (tea leaves) and proanthocyanidins (grape), have high antioxidant and anti-inflammatory activities to counteract the physiology and clinical manifestations of photoaging and photocarcinogenesis (Figure 2). The limitation has been the delivery, or targeted delivery, as well as sustained release of the polyphenols to cells (Figure 2). This limitation can be overcome through the use of polyphenols in complex with nanobiomaterials such as chitosan, liposomes, lactide-co-glycolide, and graphene nanosheets; as well as additional nanoplatforms such as phage systems (Figure 2). The goal of our laboratory would be to increase the effectiveness of xanthohumol and *P. leucotomos extract* by formulating them with these nanobiomaterials.

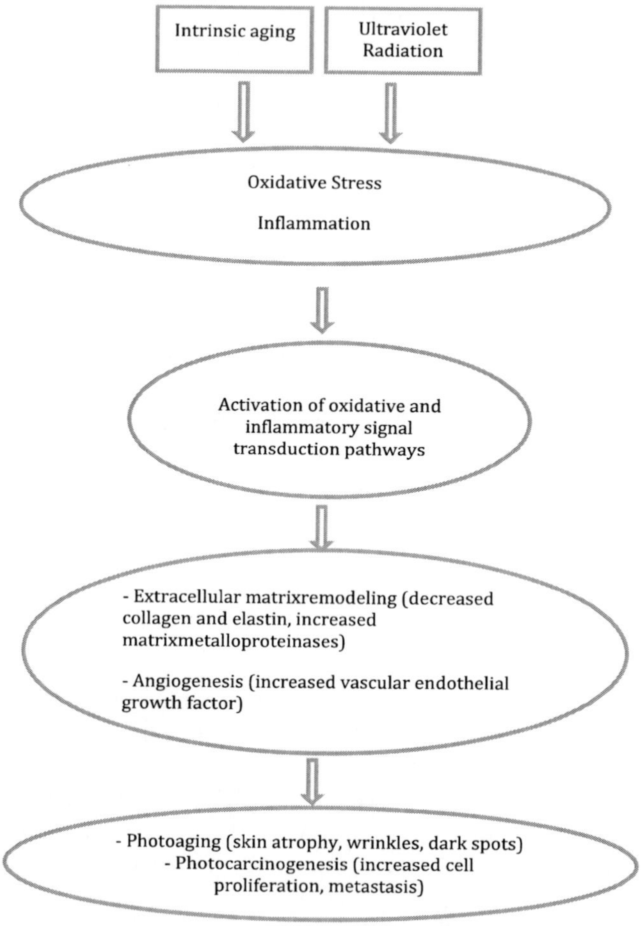

Figure 1. Mechanism of Photoaging and Photocarcinogenesis. Intrinsic factors and ultraviolet radiation induce oxidative stress and inflammation that activate signal transduction pathways to remodel the extracellular matrix.

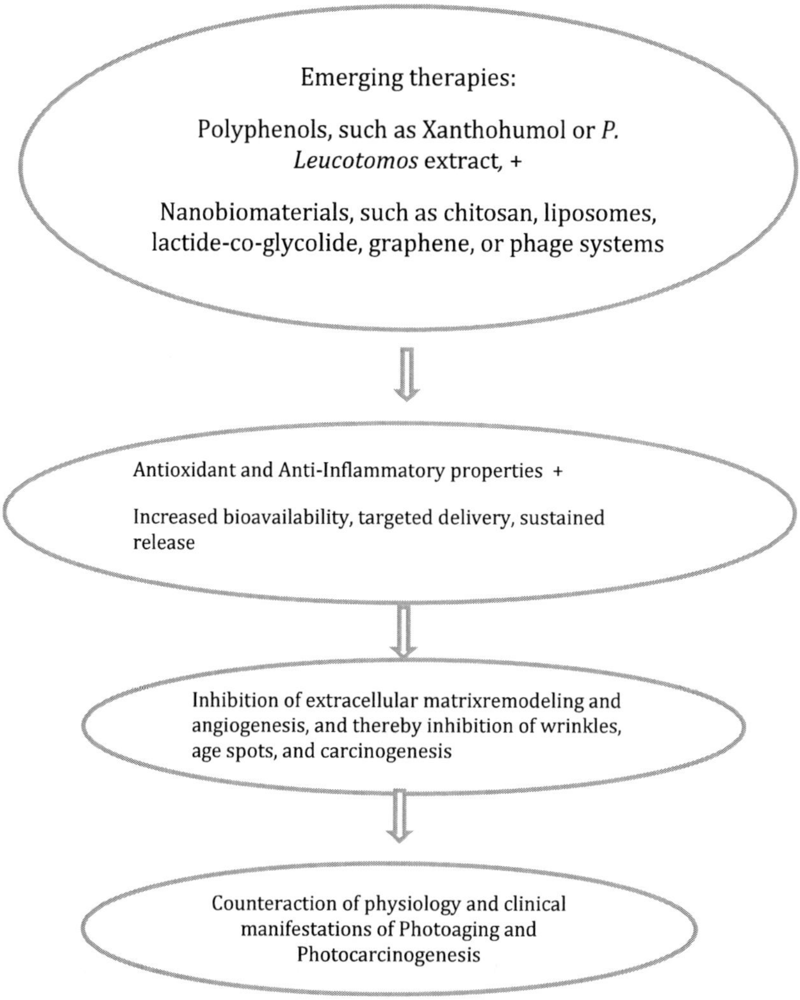

Figure 2. Counteraction of Photoaging and Photocarcinogenesis. Polyphenolic nanobiomaterial can enhance prevention of oxidative stress and inflammation to counteract photoaging and photocarcinogenesis.

References

[1] Abdolahad, M., Janmaleki, M., Mohajerzadeh, S., Akhavan, O., and Abbasi, S., 2013. Polyphenols attached graphene nanosheets for high efficiency NIR mediated photodestruction of cancer cells. *Materials Science and Engineering.* 33, 1498.

[2] Abreu, I.A., Cabelli, D.E., 2010. Superoxide dismutases-a review of the metal-associated mechanistic variations. *Biochim Biophys Acta.* 263, 74.

[3] Ahmeda, Z., Bridenb, A., Hallb, S., Brown, R.A., 2004. Stabilisation of cables of fibronectin with micromolar concentrations of copper: in vitro cell substrate properties. *Biomaterials.* 25, 803.

[4] Ahn, K.S., Moon, K.Y., Lee, J, Kim, Y.S., 2003. Downregulation of NF-kappaB activation in human keratinocytes by melanogenic inhibitors. *J Dermatol Sci.* 31,193.

[5] Ali, E.M., Sheta, M., El Mohsen, M.A., 2011. Elevated serum and tissue VEGF associated with poor outcome in breast cancer patients. *Alexandria Journal of Medicine.* 47, 217.

[6] Atsawasuwan, P., Mochida, Y., Katafuchi, M., Kaku, M., Fong, K., Csiszar, K., Yamauchi, M., 2008. Lysyl oxidase binds transforming growth factor and regulates its signaling via amine oxidase activity. *J Biol Chem.* 283, 34229.

[7] Bachelor, M.A., Bowden, G.T., 2004. UVA mediated activation of signaling pathways involved in skin tumor promotion and progression. *Semin Cancer Biol.* 14, 131.

[8] Bailey, A.J., 2001. Molecular mechanisms of ageing in connective tissues. *Mech Ageing Dev.* 122, 735.

[9] Bax, D.V., Bernard, S.E., Lomas, A., Morgan, A., Humphries, J., Shuttleworth C.A., Humphries M.J., Kielty, C.M., 2003. Cell adhesion to fibrillin-1 molecules and microfibrils is mediated by alpha(5)beta(1) and alpha(v)beta(3) integrins. *J Biol Chem.* 278, 34605.

[10] Benavente, C.A., Jacobson, M.K., Jacobson, E.L., 2009. NAD in skin: therapeutic approaches for niacin. *Current Pharmaceutical Design.*15, 29.

[11] Benavente, C.A., Jacobson, E.L., 2008. Niacin restriction upregulates NADPH oxidase and reactive oxygen species (ROS) in human keratinocytes. *Free Radic Biol Med.* 44, 527.

[12] Berg J.M., Tymoczko J.L., Stryer L., 2002. Biochemistry, 5th ed, New York, *WH Freeman.*

[13] Bissett, D.L., Oblong, J.E., and Berge, C.A., 2005. Niacinamide: A B vitamin that improves aging facial skin appearance. *Dermatol Surg.* 31, 860.

[14] Bode, W., Gomis-Rüth, F.X., Stöckler, W., 1993. Astacins, serralysins, snake venom and matrix metalloproteinases exhibit identical zinc-binding environments (HEXXHXXGXXH and Met-turn) and topologies and should be grouped into a common family, the 'metzincins'. *FEBS Lett.* 331, 134.

[15] Borkow, G., Gabbay, J., Dardik, R., Eidelman, A.I., Lavie, Y., Grunfeld, Y., Ikher, S., Huszar, M., Zatcoff, R.C., Marikovsky, M., 2010. Molecular mechanisms of enhanced wound healing by copper oxide-impregnated dressings. *Wound Repair Regen.* 18, 266.

[16] Borkow, G., Gabbay, J., Lyakhovitsky, A., Huszar, M., 2009. Improvement of facial skin characteristics using copper oxide containing pillowcases: a double-blind, placebo-controlled, parallel, randomized study. *Int J Cosmet Sci.* 31, 437.

[17] Borkow, G., Gabbay, J., Zatcoff, R.C., 2008. Could chronic wounds not heal due to too low local copper levels? *Med. Hypotheses.* 70, 610.

[18] Brennan, M., Bhatti, H., Nerusu, K.C., Bhagavathula, N., Kang, S., Fisher, G.J., Varani, J., Voorhees, J.J., 2003. Matrix metalloproteinase-1 is the major collagenolytic enzyme responsible for collagen damage in UV-irradiated human skin. *Photochem Photobiol.* 78, 43.

[19] Briganti, S., Picardo, M., 2003. Antioxidant activity, lipid peroxidation and skin diseases. What's new? Journal of the European Academy of Dermatology and Venereology. 17, 663.

[20] Callaghan, T.M., Wilhelm, K.P., 2008. A review of ageing and an examination of clinical methods in the assessment of ageing skin. Part I: Cellular and molecular perspectives of skin ageing. *Int J Cosmet Sci.* 30, 313.

[21] Carbonare, M.D., Pathak, M.A., 1992. Skin photosensitizing agents and the role of reactive oxygen species in photoaging. *J Photochem Photobiol B.* 14, 105.

[22] Chakraborti, S., Mandal, M., Das, S., Mandal, A., Chakraborti, T., 2003. Regulation of matrix metalloproteinases: an overview. *Mol Cell Biochem.* 253, 269.

[23] Cho, H.S., Lee, M.H., Lee, J.W., No, K.O., Park, S.K., Lee, H.S., Kang, S., Cho, W.G., Park, H.J., Oh, K.W., Hong, J.T., 2007. Anti-wrinkling effects of the mixture of vitamin C, vitamin E, pycnogenol and evening primrose oil, and molecular mechanisms on hairless mouse skin caused

by chronic ultraviolet B irradiation. *Photodermatol Photoimmunol Photomed.* 23, 155.

[24] Clark, L.C., Combs, G.F., Turnbull, B.W., Slate, E.H., Chalker, D.K., Chow, J., 1996. For the nutritional prevention of cancer study group. Effects of selenium supplementation for cancer prevention in patients with carcinoma of the skin. *JAMA.* 276, 1957.

[25] Colgte E.C., Miranda C.L., Stevens J.F., Bray T.M., Ho E., 2007. Xanthohumol, a prenylflavonoid derived from hops induces apoptosis and inhibits NF-kappaB activation in prostate epithelial cells. *Cancer Lett.* 246, 201.

[26] Damiani, E., Rosati, L., Castagna, R., Carloni, P., Greci, L., 2006. Changes in ultraviolet absorbance and hence in protective efficacy against lipid peroxidation of organic sunscreens after UVA irradiation. *J Photochem Photobiol B.* 82, 204.

[27] Darr, D., Pinnell, S.R., 1997. Reactive oxygen species and antioxidants protection in photodermatology. Sunscreens. (Lowe NJ, Shaat NA, Pathak MA, eds) *Marcel Dekker, Inc. 155*-173.

[28] Davis, A., Smith, G., 2002. Fallout over Disneyland. *Earth Island J.* 17, 28.

[29] Delmulle L., Bellahcène A., Dhooge W., Comhaire F., Roelens F., Huvaere K., Heyerick A., Castronovo V., De Keukeleire D., 2006. Anti-proliferative properties of prenylated flavonoids from hops (Humulus lupulus L.) in human prostate cancer cell lines. *Phytomedicine.* 13, 732.

[30] Delmulle L., Berghe T.V., Keukeleire D.D., Vandenabeele P., 2008. Treatment of PC-3 and DU145 prostate cancer cells by prenylflavonoids from hop (Humulus lupulus L.) induces a caspase-independent form of cell death. *Phytother. Res.* 22, 197

[31] Doyle, G.A., Pierce, R.A., Parks, W.C., 1997. Transcriptional induction of collagenase-1 in differentiated monocyte-like (U937) cells is regulated by AP-1 and an upstream C/EBP-β site. ***J Biol Chem.*** 272, 11840.

[32] Dwyer, J.H., Mohamed, N., Dwyer, K.M., Kholood, H., Sun, P., Shircore, A., Hama- Levy, S., 2001. Oxygenated carotenoid lutein and progression of early atherosclerosis. The Los Angeles Atherosclerosis study. *Circulation.* 103, 2922.

[33] Emanuele, E., Bertona, M., Altabas, K., Altabas, V., Alessandrini, G., 2012. Anti-inflammatory effects of a topical preparation containing nicotinamide, retinol, and 7-dehydrocholesterol in patients with acne: a gene expression study. *Clinical, Cosmetic and Invest Dermatol.* 5, 33.

[34] Felice, F., Zambito, Y., Belardinelli, E., D'Onofrio, C., Fabiano, A., Balbarini, A., Di Stefano, R., 2013. Delivery of natural polyphenols by polymeric nanoparticles improves the resistance of endothelial progenitor cells to oxidative stress. *European Journal of Pharmaceutical Sciences.* 5, 393-399

[35] Felice, F., Zambito, Y., Colo, G., D'Onofrio, C., Fausto C., 2012. Red grape skin and seeds polyphenols: Evidence of their protective effects on endothelial progenitor cells and improvement of their intestinal absorption. *Eur J Pharm Biopharm.* 80,176.

[36] Fisher, G.J., Datta, S.C., Talwar, H.S., Wang, Z.Q., Varani, J., Kang S., Voorhees J.J., 1996. Molecular basis of sun-induced premature skin ageing and retinoid antagonism. *Nature.* 379, 335.

[37] Fitzpatrick, T.B., 1988. The Validity and practicality of sun reactive skin type I-VI. *Arch Dermatol.* 124, 869.

[38] Fu, J.J, Hillebrand, G.G., Raleigh, P., Li, J., Marmor, M.J., Bertucci, V., Grimes, P.E., Mandy, S.H., Perez, M.I., Weinkle, S.H. and Kaczvinsky, J.R., 2010. A randomized, controlled comparative study of the wrinkle reduction benefits of a cosmetic niacinamide/peptide/retinyl propionate product regimen vs. a prescription 0.02% tretinoin product regimen. *Br J Dermatol.* 162, 647.

[39] Fuxe, J., Karlsson, M.C.I., 2012. TGF-β-induced epithelial-mesenchymal transition: A link between cancer and inflammation. *Seminars in Cancer Biology.* 22, 455.

[40] Gomis-Rüth, F.X., Gohlke, U., Betz, M., Knäuper, V., Murphy, G., López-Otín, C., Bode, W., 1996. The helping hand of collagenase-3 (MMP-13): 2.7 A crystal structure of its C-terminal haemopexin-like domain. *J Mol Biol.* 264, 556.

[41] Gonzalez S., Alcaraz M.V., Cuevas J., Perez M., Jaen P., Alvarex M., and Villarrubia V., 2000. An extract of the fern polypodium leucotomos (Difur®) modulates Th1/Th2 cytokines balance in vitro and appears to exhibit anti-angiogenic activities in vivo: pathogenic relationships and therapeutic implications. *Anticancer Research* 20, 1567.

[42] Gonzalez S., Pathak M.A., Cuevas J., Villarrubia V.G., and Fitzpatrick T.B., 1997. Topical or oral administration with an extract of *Polypodium leucotomos* prevents acute sunburn and psoralen-induced phototoxic reactions as well as depletion of Langerhans cells in human skin. *Photodermatol Photoimmunol Photomed.* 13, 50.

[43] Gonzalez, S., Moran, M., Kochevar, I.E., 1999. Chronic photodamage in skin of mast cell-deficient mice. *Photochem Photobiol.* 70, 248.

[44] Goodner, J., Patil, U., Lim, Y., Yarlagadda, S., Castro, A., Gonzales, S., and Philips, N., 2008. Coating on micronized titanium dioxide increases safety and maintains efficacy as sunscreen filter. *J. Plastic Dermatol.* 4, 21.

[45] Gorter, R.W., Butorac, M., Cobian, E.P., 2004. Examination of the cutaneous absorption of copper after the use of copper-containing ointments. *Am J Ther.* 11, 453.

[46] Grange, P.A., Raingeaud, J., Calvez, V., Dupin, N., 2009. Nicotinamide inhibits Propionibacterium acnes-induced IL-8 production in keratinocytes through the NF-kappaB and MAPK pathways. *J. Dermatol. Sci.* 56, 106.

[47] Guo, C., Pei-Chung Chen, Yeh, M., Hsiung, D., Wang C., 2011. Cu/Zn ratios are associated with nutritional status, oxidative stress, inflammation, and immune abnormalities in patients on peritoneal dialysis. *Clinical Biochem.* 44, 275.

[48] Herouy, Y., 2001. Matrixmetalloproteinases in skin pathology. *Int J Mol Med.* 7, 3.

[49] Hostynek, J.J., Dreher, F., Maibach, H.I., 2006. Human stratum corneum penetration by copper: In vivo study after occlusive and semi-occlusive application of the metal as powder. *Food Chem Toxicol.* 44, 1539.

[50] Hruza, L.L., Pentland, A.P., 1993. Mechanisms of UV-induced inflammation. *Invest Dermatol.* 100, 35S.

[51] Hubmacher, D., Tiedemann, K., Reinhardt, D.P., 2006. Fibrillins: from biogenesis of microfibrils to signaling functions. *Curr Top Dev Biol.*75, 93.

[52] Ingram, D., 1994. Diet and subsequent survival in women with breast cancer. *Br J Cancer.* 69, 71.

[53] Jain, M., Miller, A.B., To, T., 1994. Premorbid diet and the prognosis of women with breast cancer. *J Natl Cancer Inst.* 86, 1390.

[54] Jańczyk A., Garcia-Lopez M.A., Fernandez-Peñas P., Alonso-Lebrero J.L., Benedicto I., López-Cabrera M., and Gonzalez S., 2007. A Polypodium leucotomos extract inhibits solar-simulated radiation-induced TNF-alpha and iNOS expression, transcriptional activation and apoptosis. *Exp Dermatol.* 16, 823.

[55] Jimenez, F., Mitts, T.F., Liu, K., Wang, Y., Hinek, A., 2006. Ellagic and tannic acids protect newly synthesized elastic fibers from premature enzymatic degradation in dermal fibroblast cultures. *J. Invest Dermatol.* 126, 1272.

[56] Jin, Su-Eon., Hyo-Eon, J., and Soon-Sun, H., 2014. Targeted Delivery System of Nanobiomaterials in Anticancer Therapy: From Cells to Clinics. *BioMed Research International.* 814208. PMC.

[57] Jomova, K., Valko, M., 2011. Advances in metal-induced oxidative stress and human disease. *Toxicol.* 283, 65.

[58] Juárez, P., Guise, T.A., 2011. TGF-β in cancer and bone: Implications for treatment of bone metastases. *Bone.* 48, 23.

[59] Kamat, J.P., Devasagayam, T.P., 1996. Methylene blue plus light-induced lipid peroxidation in rat liver microsomes: inhibition by nicotinamide (vitamin B3) and other antioxidants. *Chem. Biol. Interact.* 99, 1.

[60] Kargi, A., Yalcin, A.D., Erin, N., Savas, B., Polat, H.H., Gorczynski, R.M., 2012. IL8 and serum soluble TRAIL levels following anti-VEGF monoclonal antibody treatment in patients with metastatic colon cancer. *Clin Lab.* 58, 501.

[61] Karroum, A., Mirshahi, P., Faussat, A., Therwath, A., Mirshahi, M., Hatmi, M., 2012. Tubular network formation by adriamycin-resistant MCF-7 breast cancer cells is closely linked to MMP-9 and VEGFR-2/VEGFR-3 over-expressions. *European Journal of Pharmacology.* 685,1.

[62] Kawada, A., Konishi, N., Oiso, N., Kawara, S., and Date, A., 2008. Evaluation of anti-wrinkle effects of a novel cosmetic containing niacinamide. *J. Dermatol.* 35, 637.

[63] Keeley, F.W., Bellingham, C.M., Woodhouse K.A., 2002. Elastin as a self-organizing biomaterial: use of recombinantly expressed human elastin polypeptides as a model for investigations of structure and self-assembly of elastin. *Philos Trans R Soc B Biol Sci.* 357, 185.

[64] Khorramizadeh, M.R., Tredget, E.E., Telaskyr, C., Shen, Q., Ghahary A., 1999. Aging differentially modulates the expression of collagen and collagenase in dermal fibroblasts. *Mol Cell Biochem.* 194, 99.

[65] Kielty, C.M., Sherratt, M.J., Shuttleworth, C.A., 2002. Elastic fibres. *J Cell Sci.* 115, 2817.

[66] Kielty, C.M., Woolley, D.E., Whittaker, S.P., Shuttleworth, C.A., 1994. Catabolism of intact fibrillin microfibrils by neutrophil elastase, chymotrypsin and trypsin. *FEBS Lett.* 351, 85.

[67] Kindt, T.J., Goldsby, R.A., Osborne, B.A., 2007 *Kuby Immunology.* 6th edition. *W. H. Freeman and Company.*

[68] Kinsey, R., Williamson, M.R., Chaudhry, S., Mellody, K.T., McGovern, A., Takahashi, S., Shuttleworth, C.A., Kielty, C.M., 2008. Fibrillin-1

microfibril deposition is dependent on fibronectin assembly. *J Cell Sci.* 121, 2696.

[69] Kligman, A.M., 1988. Preventing, delaying, and repairing photoaged skin. *Cutis.* 41, 419.

[70] Kligman, L.H., 1986. Photoaging. Manifestations, Prevention, and Treatment. *Dermatol Clin.* 4, 517.

[71] Kothapalli, C.R., Ramamurthi A., 2009. Copper nanoparticle cues for biomimetic cellular assembly of crosslinked elastin fibers. *Acta Biomaterialia.* 5541.

[72] Krinsky, N.I., 1994. Carotenoids and cancer: Basic research studies. In: National Antioxidants in Human health and disease. (Frei, B, ed.). *Academic press.* 239.

[73] Krutmann, J., 2001. The role of UVA rays in skin aging. *Eur J Dermatol.* 11, 170.

[74] Labat-Robert, J., Fourtanier, A., Boyer-Lafargue, B., Robert, L., 2000. Age dependent increase of elastase type protease activity in mouse skin. Effect of UV-irradiation. *J. Photochem Photobiol.* 57, 113.

[75] Lappas, M., Permezel, M., 2011. The anti-inflammatory and antioxidative effects of nicotinamide, a vitamin B (3) derivative, are elicited by FoxO3 in human gestational tissues: implications for preterm birth. *J. Nutr. Biochem.* 22, 1195.

[76] Lee, C., Choi, H., Kim, H., Kim, D., Chang, I., Moon, H.T., Lee, S., Oh, W.K., Woo, E., 2008. Biflavonoids isolated from selaginella tamariscina regulate the expression of matrix metalloproteinase in human skin fibroblasts. *Bioorg Med Chem.* 16, 732.

[77] Lemay M., Murray M.A., Davies A., Roh-Schmidt H., Randolph R., 2004. In vitro and ex vivo cyclooxygenase inhibition by a hops extract. *Asia Pac J Clin Nutr.* 13, S110.

[78] Liang X.J., 2013. Nanopharmaceutics, *Beijing, World Scientific.*

[79] Liu, D., Gharavi, R., Pitta, M., Gleichmann, M., Mattson, M.P., 2009. Nicotinamide prevents NAD+ depletion and protects neurons against excitotoxicity and cerebral ischemia: NAD+ consumption by SIRT1 may endanger energetically compromised neurons. *Neuromolecular Med.* 11, 28.

[80] Lodish, H., Berk, A., Kaiser, C.A., Krieger, M., Scott, M.P., Bretscher, A., Ploegh, H., Matsudaira, P., 2008. Molecular cell biology. 6th Edition. *W.H. Freeman and Company.*

[81] Luo Y., Eggler A.L., Liu D., Liu G., Mesecar A.D., van Breemen R.B., 2007. Sites of alkylation of human keap1 by natural chemoprevention agents. *J Am Soc Mass Spectrom.* 18, 2226.
[82] Lust S., Vanhoecke B., Janssens A., Philippe J., Bracke M., Offner F., 2005. Xanthohumol kills B-chronic lymphocytic leukemia cells by an apoptotic mechanism. *Mol Nutr Food Res.* 49, 844.
[83] Maiese, K., Chong, Z.Z., Hou, J., and Shang, Y.C., 2009. The vitamin nicotinamide: translating nutrition into clinical care. *Molecules.* 14, 3446.
[84] Maquart, F.X., Pickart, L., Laurent, M., Gillery, P., Monboisse, J.C., Borel, J.P. 1988. Glycyl-L-histidyl-L-lysine (GHK) is a tripeptide with affinity for copper (II) ions. *FEBS Lett.* 238, 343.
[85] Maquart, X., Bellon G., Chaqour, B., Wegrowski J., Leonard, M., Patt, T., Ronald, E., Trachy, Monboisse, J.C., Chastang, F., Birembaut, P., Gillery, P., Borel, J.P., 1993. In vivo stimulation of connective tissue accumulation by the tripeptide-copper complex glycyl-L-histidyl-L-lysine-Cu2+ in rat experimental wounds. *J Clin Invest.* 92, 2368.
[86] Mc Bride, Preston, P.D., Loeb, LA., 1991. Mutagenic spectrum resulting from DNA damage by Oxygen Radicals. *Biochem.* 30, 207.
[87] Mecham, R.P., Davis, E.C., 1994. Elastic fiber structure and assembly. New York*: Academic Press.*
[88] Melnikova, V.O., Ananthaswamy, H.N., 2005. Cellular and molecular events leading to the development of skin cancer. *Mutation Res.* 571, 91.
[89] Merryman, J.I., Neilsen, N., Staton, D.D., 1998. Transforming growth factor-beta enhances the ultraviolet-mediated stress response in p53-/- keratinocytes. *Int. J. Oncol.* 13, 781.
[90] Mezzeti, A., Pirdomenico, S.D., Costantini, F., Romano, F., De Cesare, D., Cuccurullo, F., Imbastaro, T., Riario-Sforza, G., Di Giacomo, F., Zuliani, G., Fellin, R., 1998. Copper/zinc ratio and systemic oxygen load: Effect of aging and aging-related degenerative diseases. *Free Radic Biol Med.* 25, 676.
[91] Millis, A.J., Hoyle, M., McCue, H.M., Martini, H., 1992. Differential expression of metalloproteinase and tissue inhibitor of metalloproteinase genes in aged human fibroblasts. *Exp Cell Res.* 201, 373.
[92] Monteiro R., Faria A., Azevedo I., Calhau C., 2007. Modulation of breast cancer cell survival by aromatase inhibiting hop (Humulus lupulus L.) flavonoids. *J Steroid Biochem Mol Biol.* 105, 124.
[93] Morera, Y., Bequet-Romero, M., Ayala, M., Velazco, J.C., Pérez, P.P., Alba, J.S., Ancizar, J., Rodríguez, M., Cosme, K., Gavilondo, J.V.,

2010. Immunogenicity and some safety features of a VEGF-based cancer therapeutic vaccine in rats, rabbits and non-human primates. *Vaccine.* 28, 3453.

[94] Morganti P., 2009. Chitin Nanofibrils in Skin Treatment. *J Appl Cosmetol.* 27, 251.

[95] Morganti P., 2010. Chitin Nanofibrils and their Derivatives as Cosmeceuticals. In SK Kim (ed): *Chitin, Chitosan, Oligosaccharides and their Derivatives. Biological Activities and Application,* New York, *CRC-Press.* pp 531.

[96] Morganti P., 2013. Innovation, Nanotechnology and Industrial Sustainability by the use of Natural Underutilized Byproducts: the EU support to SMEs, *Journal of Molecular Biochemistry.* 2, 137.

[97] Morganti P., Del Ciotto P., and Gao C.H., 2012. Skin Delivery and Controlled release of Active ingredients nanoencapsulated. *Cosmetic Science Technology.* 20, 136.

[98] Morganti P., Di Massimo G.,, Cimini C., and Del Ciotto P., 2013. Characterization of Chitin nanofibrill-Hyaluronan Block Polymer *Personal Care.* 6, 61.

[99] Nagase, H., Woessner, J.F., 1999. Matrix Metalloproteinases. *J Biol Chem.* 274, 21491.

[100] Nichols, J.A., Katiyar, S.K., 2010. Skin photoprotection by natural polyphenols: anti-inflammatory, antioxidant and DNA repair mechanisms. *Arch Dermatol Res.* 302, 71.

[101] O'Rourke, M.F., Hashimoto, J. 2007. Mechanical factors in arterial aging: a clinical perspective. *J Am Coll Cardiol.* 50, 1.

[102] Perelshtein, I., Ruderman, E., Francesko, A., Fernandes, M., Tzanov, T., Gedanken, A., 2014. Tannic acid NPs – Synthesis and immobilization onto a solid surface in a one-step process and their antibacterial and anti-inflammatory properties. *Ultrasonics Sonochemistry.* 21, 1916-1920

[103] Perrot, C., Javelaud, D., Mauviel, A., 2012. Overlapping activities of TGF-β and hedgehog signaling in cancer: Therapeutic targets for cancer treatment. *Pharmacology & Therapeutic.* Available online.

[104] Philips N., Smith J., Keller T., Gonzalez S., 2003. Predominant effects of Polypodium leucotomos on membrane integrity, lipid peroxidation, and expression of elastin and matrixmetalloproteinase-1 in ultraviolet radiation exposed fibroblasts, and keratinocytes. *J Dermatol Sci.* 32, 1.

[105] Philips, N., 2003. An anti TGF-β increased the expression of transforming growth factor-β, matrix metallproteinase-1 and elastin, and

its effects were antagonized by ultraviolet radiation in epidermal keratinocytes. *J. Dermatol. Sci.* 33, 177.

[106] Philips, N., Burchill, D., O'Donoghue, D., Keller, T., and Gonzalez, S., 2004a. Identification of benzene metabolites in dermal fibroblasts: Regulation of cell viability, apoptosis, lipid peroxidation, and expression of MMP-1 and elastin by benzene metabolites. *Skin Pharmacol and Physiol.* 17, 147.

[107] Philips, N., Devaney, J., 2004b. Beneficial regulation of type I collagen and matrixmetalloproteinase –1 expression by estrogen, progesterone, and its combination in skin fibroblasts. *J Am Aging Association.* 26, 59.

[108] Philips, N., Keller, T., Hendrix, C., Hamilton, S., Arena, R., Tuason, M., Gonzalez, S., 2007. Regulation of the extracellular matrix remodeling by lutein in dermal fibroblasts, melanoma cells, and ultraviolet radiation exposed fibroblasts. *Arch Dermatol Res.* 299, 373.

[109] Philips, N., Keller, T., Hendrix, C., Hamilton, S., Arena, R., Tuason, M., Gonzalez, S., 2007a. Regulation of the extracellular matrix remodeling by lutein in dermal fibroblasts, melanoma cells, and ultraviolet radiation exposed fibroblasts. *Arch Dermatol Res.* 299, 373.

[110] Philips, N., Keller, T., Holmes, C., 2007b. Reciprocal effects of ascorbate on cancer cell growth and the expression of matrix metalloproteinases and transforming growth factor-beta. *Cancer Letters.* 256, 49.

[111] Philips N., Dulaj L., Upadhya T., 2009. Growth inhibitory mechanism of ascorbate and counteraction of its matrix metalloproteinases-1 and transforming growth factor-beta stimulation by gene silencing or *P. leucotomos. Anti Cancer Res.* 29, 3233.

[112] Philips, N., Conte, J., Chen, Y., Natrajan, P., Taw, M., Keller, T., Givant, J., Tuason, M., Dulaj, L., Leonardi, D., Gonzalez, S., 2009a. Beneficial regulation of matrixmetalloproteinases and its inhibitors, fibrillar collagens and transforming growth factor-β by P. leucotomos, directly or in dermal fibroblasts, ultraviolet radiated fibroblasts, and melanoma cells. *Arch Derm Res.* 301, 487.

[113] Philips, N., Tuason, M., Chang, T., Lin, Y., Tahir, M., Rodriguez, S.G., 2009b. Differential effects of ceramide on cell viability and extracellular matrix remodeling in keratinocytes and fibroblasts. *Skin Pharmacol Physiol.* 22, 151.

[114] Philips, N., Arena, R., Yarlagadda, S., 2009c. Inhibition of ultraviolet radiation mediated extracellular matrix remodeling in fibroblasts by transforming growth factor-β. *BIOS.* 80, 1.

[115] Philips, N., Hwang, H., Chauhan, S., Leonardi, D., Gonzalez, S., 2010a. Stimulation of cell proliferation, and expression of matrixmetalloproteinase-1 and interluekin-8 genes in dermal fibroblasts by copper. *Connective Tissue Res.* 51, 224.

[116] Philips, N., Samuel, M., Arena, R., Chen, Y., Conte, J., Natrajan, P., Haas, G., Gonzalez, S., 2010b. Direct inhibition of elastase and matrixmetalloproteinases, and stimulation of biosynthesis of fibrillar collagens, elastin and fibrillins by xanthohumol. *J Cosmet Sci.* 61, 125.

[117] Philips, N., Samuel, P., Parakandi, H., Gopal, S., Siomyk, H., Ministro, A., Thompson, T., Borkow, G., 2012. Beneficial regulation of fibrillar collagens, heat shock protein-47, elastin fiber components, transforming growth factor-β1 vascular endothelial growth factor and oxidative stress effects by copper in dermal fibroblasts. *Connective Tissue Res.*

[118] Philips, N., Siomyk, H., Bynum, D., Gonzalez, S., 2013. Skin Cancer, polyphenols, and oxidative Stress. In Cancer: Oxidative Stress and Dietary Antioxidants, Kings College London, *Elsevier.*

[119] Pickart, L., 2008. The human tri-peptide GHK and tissue remodeling. *J Biomater Sci Polym Ed.* 19, 969.

[120] Pinkas-Sarafova, A., Markova, N.G., Simon, M., 2005. Dynamic changes in nicotinamide pyridine dinucleotide content in normal human epidermal keratinocytes and their effect on retinoic acid biosynthesis. *Biochemical and Biophys Res Commun.* 336, 554.

[121] Preston, D., Stern, R.S., 1992. Non melanoma skin cancer of the skin. *N Engl J Med* 327, 1649.

[122] Qin, Y., Wang, H., Karuppanapandian, T., Wook, K., 2010. Chitosan green tea polyphenol complex as a released control compound for wound healing. *Chin J Traumatol.* 13, 91.

[123] Qin, Y., Xing, G., Li, L., Wang, H., Wook, K, 2013. The antioxidant property of chitosan green tea polyphenols complex induces transglutaminase activation in wound healing. *J Med Food.* 16, 487.

[124] Ramirez, F., Pereira, L., 1999. The fibrillins. *Int J Biochem Cell Biol.* 31, 255.

[125] Ratner B.D., Hoffman A.S., Schoen F.J., 2004. Biomaterials Science:An Introduction to Materials in Medicine. 2nd Edition. New York, *Academic Press.*

[126] Robert, L., 2002. Elastin, past, present and future. *Pathol Biol.* 50, 503.

[127] Robert, L., Robert, A.M., Fulop, T., 2008. Rapid increase in human life expectancy: will it soon be limited by the aging of elastin? *Biogerontology.* 9, 119.

[128] Rock, M.J., Cain, S.A., Freeman, L.J., Morgan, A., Mellody, K., Marson, A., Shuttleworth, C.A., Weiss, A.S., Kielty, C.M., 2004. Molecular basis of elastic fiber formation: critical interactions and a tropoelastin-fibrillin-1 cross-link. *J Biol Chem.* 279, 23748.

[129] Rosen Y., Elman N., Horowitz E., 2012. Introduction. In Y Rosen and N. Elman (Eds) Biomaterial Science.An integraded Clinical and Engineering Approach, Boca Raton (Fl) CRC-Press. pp1.

[130] Rucker, R.B., Kosonen, T., Clegg, M.S., Mitchell, A.E., Rucker, B.R., Uriu-Hare, J.Y., Keen, C.L., 1998. Copper lysyl oxidase, and extracellular matrix protein cross-linking. *Am J Clin Nutr.* 67, 996S.

[131] Sandler, A., Hirsh, V., Reck, M., von Pawel, J., Akerley, W., Johnson, D.H., 2012. An evidence-based review of the incidence of CNS bleeding with anti-VEGF therapy in non-small cell lung cancer patients with brain metastases. *Lung Cancer.* 78, 1.

[132] Schiff, K., Brown, J., Diehl, D., Greenstein, D., 2007. Extent and magnitude of copper contamination in the marinas of San Diego region, California, USA. *Marine Pollution Bull.* 54, 322.

[133] Shin J., Shin K., Lee H., Nam J.B., Jung J.E., Ryu J.H., Han J.H. et al., 2010. Non-invasive transdermal Delivery Route Using Electrostatically Interactive Biocompatible Nanocapsules. *Adv Mater.* 22, 739.

[134] Siméon, A., Emonard, H., Hornebeck, W., Maquart, F.X., 2000. Thc tripeptide-copper complex glycyl-L-histidyl-L- lysine-Cu2+ stimulates matrix metalloproteinase-2 expression by fibroblast cultures. *Life Sci.* 67, 2257.

[135] Sims, T.J., Rasmussen, L.M., Oxlund, H., Bailey, A.J., 1996. The role of glycation cross-links in diabetic vascular stiffening. *Diabetologia.* 39, 946.

[136] Smith, G., 2000. Fireworks and pollution. *Earth Island J.* 15, 28.

[137] Smith-Mungo, L, Kagan H., 1998. Lysyl oxidase: properties, regulation and multiple functions in biology. *Matrix Biol.* 16, 387.

[138] Srivastava, A., 2013. Synthesis of PLGA Nanoparticles of Tea Polyphenols and Their Strong in Vivo Protective Effect Against Chemically Induced DNA Damage. *International Journal of Nanomedicine.* 8, 1451.

[139] Surjana, D., Halliday, G.M., Damian, D.L., 2010. Role of nicotinamide in DNA damage, mutagenesis, and DNA repair. *J Nucleic Acids.*

[140] Svobodova, A., Walterova. D., Vostalova., 2006. Ultraviolet light induced alteration to the skin. *Biomed Pap Med Fac Univ Palacky Olomouc Czech Repub.* 150, 25.

[141] Szauter, K.M., Cao, T., Boyd, C.D., Csiszar, K., 2005. Lysyl oxidase in development, aging and pathologies of the skin. *Pathol Biol.* 53, 448.

[142] Toyoda, M., Bhawan, J., 1995. Electron-microscopic observations of cutaneous photoaging versus intrinsic aging. *J Geriatr Dermatol.* 3,131.

[143] Tsuji, N., Moriwaki, S., Suzuki, Y., Takema, Y., Imokawa, G., 2001. The role of elastases secreted by fibroblasts in wrinkle formation: implication through selective inhibition of elastase activity. *Photochem Photobiol.* 71, 283.

[144] Ushio-Fukai M., 2006. Redox signaling in angiogenesis: Role of NADPH oxidase. *Cardiovascular research* 71, 226.

[145] Ushio-Fukai M., and Nakamura Y., 2008. Reactive oxygen species and angiogenesis: NADPH oxidase as target for cancer therapy. *Cancer letters* 266, 37.

[146] Van Wart, H.E., Birkedal-Hansen, H., 1990. The cysteine switch: a principle of regulation of metalloproteinase activity with potential applicability to the entire matrix metalloproteinase gene family. *Proc Natl Acad Sci.* 87, 5578.

[147] Vanhoecke B., Derycke L., Van Marck V., Depypere H., De Keukeleire D., Bracke M., 2005. Antiinvasive effect of xanthohumol, a prenylated chalcone present in hops (Humulus lupulus L.) and beer. *Int J Cancer.* 117, 889.

[148] Verstappen, J., Von den Hoff, J.W., 2006. Tissue Inhibitors of Metalloproteinases (TIMPs): Their Biological Functions and Involvement in Oral Diseases. *Crit Rev Oral Biol Med J Dent Res.* 85, 1074.

[149] Vile, G.F., Tanew-Iliitschew, A., Tyrrell, R.M., 2008. Activation of NF-KB in human skin fibroblasts by the oxidative stress generated by UVA radiation. *Photochemistry and Photobiol.* 62, 463.

[150] Viquez, O.M., Holly, L. Valentine, Kalyani Amarnath, Dejan Milatovic, William M. Valentine., 2008. Copper accumulation and lipid oxidation precede inflammation and myelin lesions in N, N-diethyldithiocarbamate peripheral myelinopathy. *Toxicol and Applied Pharmacol.* 229, 77.

[151] Voruganti, V.S., Klein, G.L., Lu, H.X., Thomas, S., Freeland-Graves, J.H., Herndon, D.N., 2005. Impaired zinc and copper status in children with burn injuries: Need to reassess nutritional requirements. *Burns.* 31, 711.

[152] Wang, B., Kaumaya, P.T.P., Cohn, D.E., 2010. Immunization with synthetic VEGF peptides in ovarian cancer. *Gynecologic Oncology.* 119, 564.

[153] Watson, R.E., Craven, N.M., Kang, S., Jones, C.J., Kielty, C.M., Griffits, C.E., 2001. A short-term screening protocol, using fibrillin-1 as a reporter molecule, for photoaging repair agents. *J Invest Dermatol.* 116, 672.

[154] Watson, R.E., Griffits, C.E., Craven, N.M., Shuttleworth, C.A., Kielty, C.M., 1999. Fibrillin-rich microfibrils are reduced in photoaged skin. Distribution at the dermal-epidermal junction. *J Invest Dermatol.* 112, 782.

[155] Wlaschek, M., Tantcheva-Poór I., Naderi L., Ma W., Schneider L.A., Razi-Wolf Z., Schüller J., Scharffetter-Kochanek K., 2001. Solar UV irradiation and dermal photoaging. *J Photochem Photobiol B.* 63, 41.

[156] Yaar, M., Gilchrest, B.A., 2007. Photoageing: mechanism, prevention and therapy. *Br J Dermatol.* 157, 874.

[157] Yan, C., Boyd, D.D., 2007. Regulation of matrix metalloproteinase gene expression. *J Cell Physiol.* 211, 19.

[158] Yang J.Y., Della-Fera M.A., Rayalam S., Baile C.A., 2007. Effect of xanthohumol and isoxanthohumol on 3T3-L1 cell apoptosis and adipogenesis. *Apoptosis.* 12, 1953.

[159] Yang, L., You, S., Kumar, V., Zhang, C., Cao, Y., 2012. In vitro the behaviors of metastasis with suppression of VEGF in human bone metastatic LNCaP-derivative C4-2B prostate cancer cell linc. *J Exp Clin Cancer Res.* 31, 40.

[160] Zhang, H., Hu, W., Ramirez, F., 1995. Developmental expression of fibrillin genes suggests heterogeneity of extracellular microfibrils. *J Cell Biol.* 129, 1165.

[161] Zou, LQ., Liu, W., Liu, WL., Liang, RH., Li, T., Liu, CM., Cao, YL., Niu, J., and Liu, Z.. 2014.Characterization and bioavailability of tea polyphenol nanoliposome prepared by combining an ethanol injectionmethod with dynamic high-pressure microfluidization. *J Agric Food Chem.* 29;62, 934-41

[162] Zuo, X., Xie, H., Dong, D., Jiang, N., Zhu, H., Kang, Y.J., 2010. Cytochrome c oxidase is essential for copper-induced regression of cardiomyocyte hypertrophy. *Cardiovasc Toxicol.* 10, 208.

In: Skin Aging and Photoaging
Editor: Emanuel Graham

ISBN: 978-1-63482-907-6

Chapter 7

Ultraviolet-Induced Photoaging in the Skin: The role of Inflammatory Cytokine, Macrophage Migration Inhibitory Factor

Mati Ur Rehman[1,2], Takashi Kondo[2] and Tadamichi Shimizu[1,*]
[1]Department of Dermatology,
[2]Department of Radiological Sciences, Graduate School of Medicine and Pharmaceutical Sciences, University of Toyama, Sugitani, Toyama, Japan

Abstract

The human Skin is continuously challenged by different adverse influences such as solar radiation, chemicals and oxidative stress. The most common cause of physical injury to the skin is solar ultraviolet (UV) irradiation, which causes long-term detrimental effects, such as

* Corresponding author: Prof. Tadamichi Shimizu, M.D., Ph.D., Department of Dermatology, Graduate School of Medicine and Pharmaceutical Sciences, University of Toyama, 2630 Sugitani, Toyama 930-0194, Japan, TEL: +81-76-434-7305; FAX: +81-76-434-5190; E-mail: shimizut@med.u-toyama.ac.jp.

cutaneous photoaging. Photoaged skin is clinically characterized by wrinkles, laxity, coarseness, and the loss of skin tone and biochemically characterized by a predominance of abnormal elastic fibers in the dermis and a dramatic decrease in specific collagen types. Ultraviolet radiation induced changes in the dermal extracellular matrix proteins; the accumulation of disorganized elastin and the loss of interstitial collagens are also thought to be responsible for photo damage of the skin. Chronic skin exposure to ultraviolet radiation stimulates the production of cytokines known to play a key role in the process of photoaging and initiation of skin cancer. Macrophage migration inhibitory factor (MIF) has long been considered to be a lymphokine that concentrates macrophages at inflammatory loci, and it is a potent activator of macrophages *in vivo*, which are considered to play an important role in cell-mediated immunity. Subsequently, MIF was reevaluated and described to be a pro-inflammatory cytokine and pituitary-derived hormone that potentiates endotoxemia. MIF is expressed in the epidermis of the skin, particularly in the basal layer, and enhanced MIF production is observed in the skin after UV irradiation. This chapter will focus on the biological effects and the latest findings on the role of MIF in photoaging following UV exposure.

Keywords: Skin, cytokine, macrophage migration inhibitory factor, photoaging, ultraviolet irradiation

Introduction

The skin is the outermost layer of the body that is constantly exposed to hazards such as solar radiation, chemical challenges and oxidative stress. Among these, solar ultraviolet irradiation (UV) is the most important and common cause of skin injury. The UV is sub-divided into three types according to the wavelengths: long-wave UVA (320-400 nm), mid-wave UVB (280-320 nm) and short-wave UVC (200-280 nm). Most UVC are absorbed by the ozone layer, however, UVA and UVB radiation reaches the surface of the earth and thus causes different skin disorders [1]. Recent depletion of the stratospheric ozone has led to an increased risk for skin damage due to enhanced UVA irradiation and penetration of UVB [2]. Because the skin comes in direct contact with the environment, exposure to UV irradiation causes various adverse effects including edema, sunburn cells, hyperplasia, immunosuppression, photoaging and the development of skin cancers [3, 4].

Generally, the aging process of the skin is divided into intrinsic and extrinsic aging (photoaging). Extrinsic aging occurs mainly due to repeated UV exposure from the sun and is considered to be a different entity than the damage which occurs over the passage of time (chronologic aging), as this typically occurs in other organs of the body. Chronologically aged skin is characterized as smooth, pale and finely wrinkled. In contrast, photoaged skin is characterized by coarse wrinkles, laxity, dyspigmentation, leathery appearance, roughness and telangiectasia. Photoaging affects various skin layers, however, the major histological differences and damage occur within the dermis [5, 6, 7]. In addition, UVB radiation to skin can cause DNA damage directly or indirectly. UVB can cause direct damage to DNA and lead to the formation of cyclobutane pyrimidine dimers (CPDs) and pyrimidine (6-4) pyrimidone photoproducts (6-4 PPs), which are main photolesions in genomic DNA [8]. Moreover, UVB can also cause indirect damage to DNA through the induction of reactive oxygen species (ROS) production, thereby facilitating DNA oxidation [9, 10]. Most of the damaging UVB radiation is absorbed by the epidermis, and leads to massive apoptosis of keratinocytes, suppression of the immune system and compromises the natural barrier functions of the skin [11]. Furthermore, UV radiation may also trigger the cutaneous inflammatory response and stimulate the release of cytokines, which are known to play a crucial role in the photoaging process. Among these, one such important cytokine is macrophage migration inhibitory factor (MIF).

UV-Induced Inflammatory Cytokines in the Skin

UVB radiation is biologically very active and mostly penetrates the epidermis and, to a lesser extent, the upper part of dermis. Therefore, epidermal cells are considered to be the main target for UVB radiation. UV radiation stimulates and activates nearly all nucleated cells, such as keratinocytes and melanocytes, Langerhans cells in the epidermis and cells in dermis, such as fibroblasts, endothelial cells, and mast cells, to induce the production of various cytokines [12]. It has been known that UV radiation triggers the cutaneous inflammatory response through the stimulation of epidermal keratinocytes with the concurrent release of potent cytokines such as interleukin (IL)-1 [13, 14], IL-6 [15], and tumor necrosis factor (TNF)-α [16]. TNF-α, which is an important component of the inflammatory cascade in the skin, can affects various cell types once activated [17]. It increases MHC class I expression on endothelial cells and dermal fibroblasts; induces the production of IL-1α [18]; increases the expression of adhesion molecules, including ICAM-1, VCAM-1 and E-selectin; and promotes the formation of sunburn cells [19].

It has been known that dermal alterations due to photoaging induced by UV radiation can be mainly seen in the dermis, with massive accumulation of elastotic material in the upper and mid dermis, which is referred to as "solar elastosis". The UV-induced dermal alterations, which include elastosis and changes in collagens, are thought to be dependent on the growth and differentiation of dermal fibroblasts and are regulated by different factors including cytokines released from epidermal and infiltrating cells as well as from fibroblasts in an autocrine and paracrine manner. There is emerging evidence that growth-regulated cytokines from fibroblasts, such as TGF-α, TGF-β, PDGF, FGF, IL-1, IL-6, and TNF-α, can play a role in the control of connective tissue formation and remodeling phases of dermal fibrotic repair [12, 20]. Therefore, these cytokines are of great importance in the course of photoaging and are involved not only in the mediation of local inflammatory reactions within the skin, but can also exert systemic effects through entrance into the circulation.

UV-Induced Reactive Oxygen Species in the Skin

There is growing evidence that UV radiation significantly increases ROS generation in the skin, such as singlet oxygen, superoxide radicals, hydroxyl radicals, and hydrogen peroxide [21], and this intracellular increase in ROS is responsible for the initiation of several inflammatory responses in the skin. The skin is equipped with a complex defense system of enzymatic and non-enzymatic components to counter the adverse biological effects of ROS. As the first line of defense, ROS are reduced by antioxidant enzymes, such as superoxide dismutase (SOD), catalase, and glutathione peroxidase, as well as endogenous and exogenous small molecules, including glutathione, vitamin C and vitamin E. When the biomolecules are oxidized, they are repaired or replaced by biological protective systems. ROS are also generated as a part of normal regulatory circuits; under normal conditions the cellular redox state is tightly regulated by the antioxidant defense system of the skin, while in situations such as UV exposure, increased ROS generation can overwhelm the antioxidant defense mechanism, resulting in oxidative stress and oxidative damage to lipids, proteins and DNA, eventually leading to age-related diseases and photoaging of the skin [22, 23, 24].

UV-induced ROS generation can promote photoaging and carcinogenesis via the regulation of different molecular and signaling pathways, which has been reported in previous studies [25, 26]. In particular, UV-induced ROS generation has also been shown to stimulate the synthesis of matrix metalloproteases (MMPs) [27]. MMPs play an important role in the aging process of the skin by targeting connective tissue molecules and basement membrane proteins. Interestingly, ROS are also able to inactivate a special class of tissue inhibitors of metalloproteases (TIMPS) via a direct oxidative attack, and thus contribute in the progression of photoaging and tumor [28]. Accordingly, research has been focused on the use of antioxidants for the prevention of ROS mediated photoaging and photocarcinogenesis [29, 30]. Similarly, we have shown that SOD/catalase mimetic platinum nanoparticles (nano-Pt) are effective in reducing UV-induced ROS and apoptosis and that topically applied nano-Pt effectively protects against UV-induced skin inflammation and photoallergy [31] (Figure 1).

Macrophage Migration Inhibitory Factor (MIF)

MIF was originally identified in 1966 as a lymphokine that concentrates macrophages at inflammatory loci. It is a known potent activator of macrophages *in vivo* and is considered to play a key role in cell-mediated immunity [32, 33]. In 1989, following the molecular cloning of MIF cDNA [34], MIF was reevaluated and described as a pro-inflammatory cytokine and pituitary-derived hormone that potentiates endotoxemia [35]. With progressive research, MIF was found to be multifunctional (Figure 2), and subsequent work has shown that T cells and macrophages secrete MIF in response to glucocorticoids as well as upon activation by various pro-inflammatory stimuli [36]. MIF plays a role as a pleiotropic cytokine by participating in inflammation and immune responses [37]. The expression of MIF is increased in many solid tumors [38, 39], and in several cases the degree of MIF overexpression is strongly correlated with tumor progression and metastatic potential. MIF additionally plays a key role in cell proliferation and invasion

[40, 41]. Furthermore, MIF has broader effects on glucocorticoid-induced immunomodulation [42], D-dopachrome tautomerase activity [43], innate immunity relevance to Toll-like receptor 4 [44] and is a crucial effector of hypoxia-inducible factor 1α which delays senescence [45]. It has been reported that MIF is expressed primarily in T cells and macrophages; however, more recent studies have shown that this protein is ubiquitously expressed by many cell types, indicating a more extensive non-immunological involvement in a variety of pathological states [37, 46]. In addition, a potentially broader role for MIF is reported in growth regulation due to its ability to antagonize p53-mediated gene activation and apoptosis [47].

In the skin, MIF is expressed in the epidermis, particularly in the basal layer [48]. MIF is responsible for important implications in the skin with regard to inflammation, the immune response, and cutaneous wound healings and also plays a crucial role in skin diseases, such as atopic dermatitis and systemic lupus erythematosus [49].

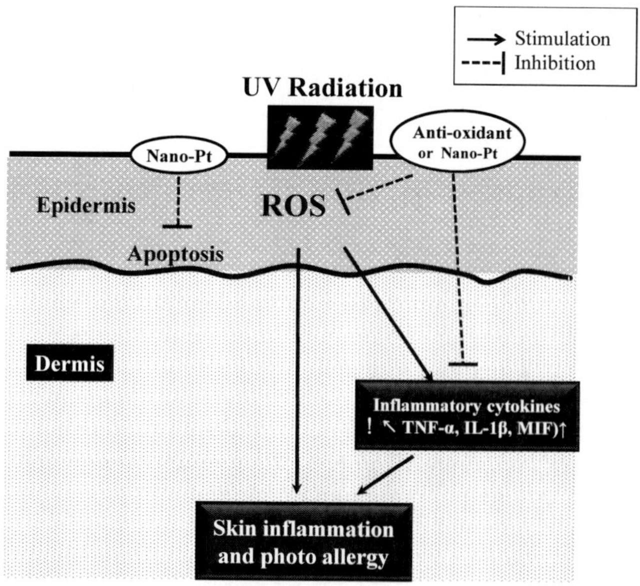

Figure 1. A schematic diagram of the protective effects of antioxidants or SOD/ catalase mimetic platinum nanoparticles against UV-induced ROS mediated inflammatory cytokines production and skin inflammation.

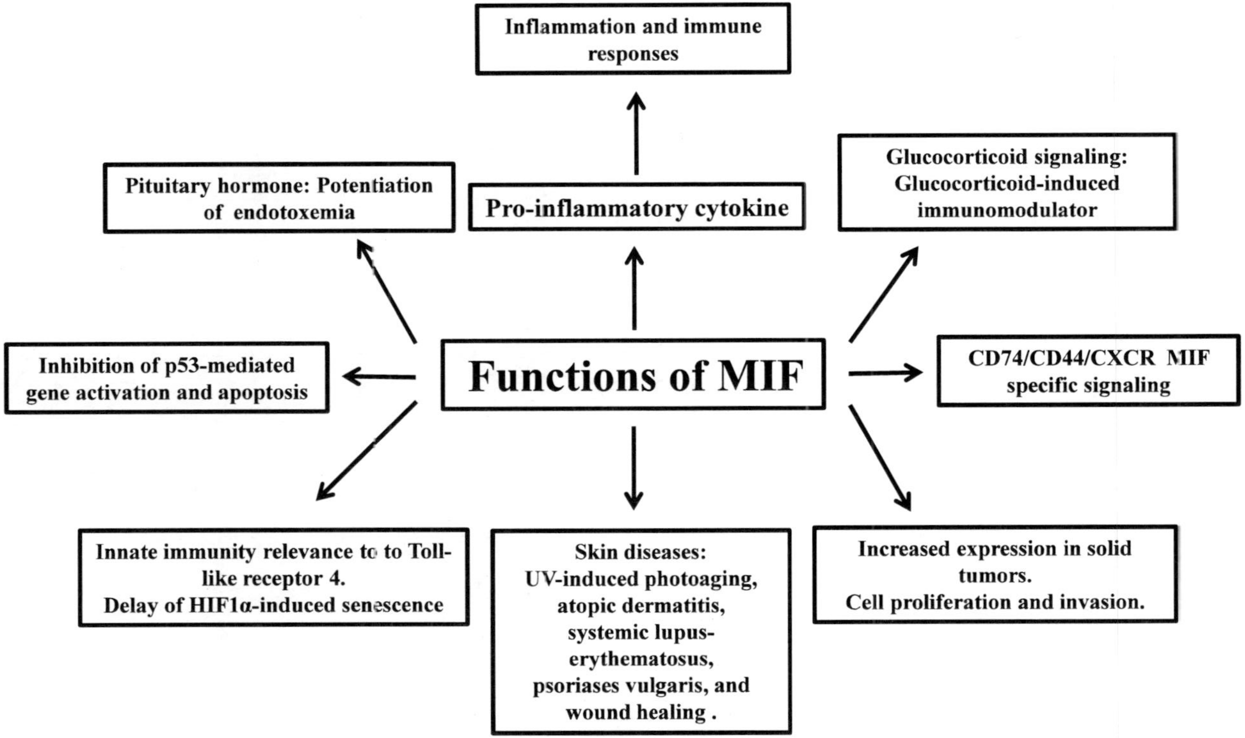

Figure 2. A schematic diagram of the multiple functions of macrophage migration inhibitory factor (MIF).

UV-Induced Photoaging in the Skin: The Role of MIF

Acute UV exposure has various deleterious cutaneous effects in the skin, including edema, sunburn cells, hyperplasia, the production of inflammatory mediators and immunosuppression. The long-term detrimental effects of repeated UV exposure lead to cutaneous photoaging or skin cancer. Skin cancer, which is the most prevalent form of cancer in humans, most commonly occurs in photoaged skin. Photoaged skin is clinically characterized by wrinkles, laxity, coarseness, and the loss of skin tone and biochemically characterized by a predominance of abnormal elastic fibers in the dermis and a dramatic decrease in specific collagen types. Interstitial collagens, the major structural components of the dermis, are particularly reduced in UV-irradiated actinically damaged skin [50, 51, 52]. The MMP family is still being discovered, however, it is known to play a crucial role in tissue destruction during pathological conditions, such as arthritis, skin aging, tumor invasion, and metastasis [53]. Growing evidence clearly indicates the occurrence of several morphological and biochemical indicators, which suggest that the amount and normal structure of collagen type I is reduced in UV-damaged skin [54]. Some MMPs, such as MMP-1, play a major role in the photoaging process while others, such as MMP-2 and MMP-9, potently promote the degradation of collagen type IV, a major component of the basement membrane. The reduction of collagen type IV at the dermal-epidermal junction has been associated with wrinkling skin [55].

UV-induced MMPs, present in keratinocytes and dermal fibroblasts, are known to contribute to the breakdown of dermal interstitial collagen and other connective tissue components. This skin damage mechanism involves a number of secreted cytokines, including interleukin (IL)-1, IL-6 and TNF-α [13, 14, 15, 16]. Along with these cytokines, previous studies conducted in our laboratory have shown that UV also enhances the production of MIF in the skin, and both UVA and UVB were found to increase the expression of MIF in human dermal fibroblasts and epidermal keratinocytes, respectively [56, 57]. Recently, MIF was also found to be involved in the basement membrane damage in chronically UVB-exposed skin in mice. MIF mRNA and protein levels were significantly increased in UVB-irradiated skin in MIF Tg mice. This increase in MIF production was also correlated with the UVB-induced upregulation of MMP-2 and MMP-9, whereas it resulted in diminished levels of type IV collagen. In addition, when the effects of MIF were inhibited using a specific MIF inhibitor ISO-1, the UVB-induced mRNA levels and the production of MMP-9 in keratinocytes and MMP-2 in fibroblasts were also suppressed [58]. Therefore, it is quite evident that MIF plays a key role in collagen degradation and basement membrane damage, which occurs primarily through the activation of MMP-9 and MMP-2. In addition, MIF upregulates the activity of MMP-1 and is also involved in the activation of UVA-induced MMP-1 in dermal fibroblasts. This MIF-mediated MMP-1 activation in dermal fibroblasts is dependent on the MIF-induced stimulation of PKC-, PKA-, Src-family tyrosine kinase, MAPK-, c-Jun- and AP-1-dependent pathways [57]. Moreover, previously a study showed that IL-1β is also involved in the upregulation of UVA-induced MMP-1 in dermal fibroblasts through p38-, JNK- and PKC-dependent pathways [59]. It is clear that the signal-transduction pathways involved in IL-1β or MIF-induced MMP-1 in dermal fibroblasts are different. Interestingly, IL-1β stimulation itself causes a significant increase in specific MIF mRNA and protein levels in human dermal fibroblasts, while MIF is unable to stimulate IL-1β expression and production in dermal fibroblast. Furthermore, neutralizing the effects of MIF with anti-MIF antibody also suppresses the MMP-1 expression induced by IL-1β. Therefore, UVA radiation may lead to IL-1β-induced MMP-1 expression and IL-1β-mediated MIF stimulation also enhances the MMP-1 expression in dermal fibroblasts. Dermal fibroblasts from MIF-deficient mice showed much less sensitivity to IL-1β-induced MMP-13 production, although MMP-13 is not very prominent in human tissues and plays a limited role. It is mainly believed to act as a tissue collagenase in rodents [59]. Therefore, there is great possibility that IL-1β may stimulate MMP-13 production via MIF in dermal fibroblasts. Taken together, these findings strongly suggest that in fibroblasts UVA radiation may stimulate IL-1β production via an autocrine loop of both IL-1β and MIF. Thus, both IL-1β and MIF have roles in the synthesis of MMP-1 (MMP-13). Furthermore, MIF has been shown to be involved in the induction of granzyme B (GrB) after UVA-radiation. UVA induces a redox-dependent release of MIF, which, in turn, activates the production of active GrB through the p38 MAPK pathway [60]. GrB induction by UVA was able to degrade fibronectin. Taken together, these studies suggest that MIF is a key modulator of MMPs, such as MMP-1, MMP-2, MMP-9, and granzyme B after UV radiation (Figure 3).

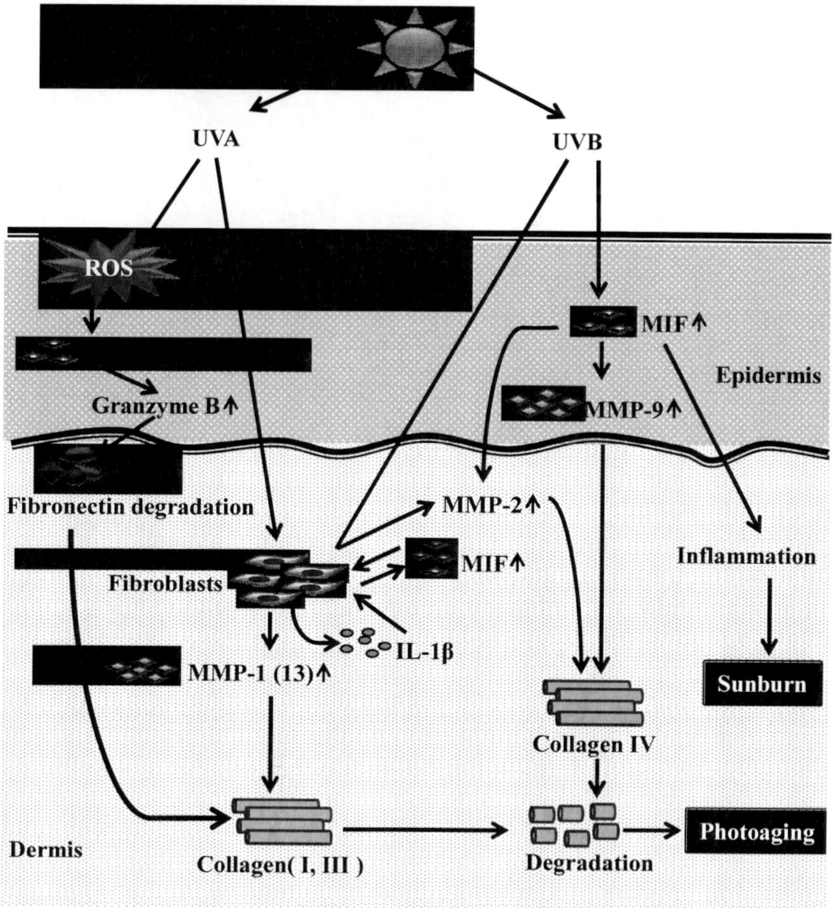

Figure 3. A schematic illustration of MIF-related photoaging. UV radiation, including both UVA and UVB, leads to the increased secretion of MIF by keratinocytes and fibroblasts, respectively. MIF increases the UVB-induced MMPs expression, particularly MMP-2 in fibroblasts and MMP-9 in keratinocytes, which subsequently contributes to MIF-mediated basement membrane damage and collagen degradation, specifically collagen IV. Chronic UVA radiation stimulates MIF production in dermal fibroblasts through an autocrine loop involving both MIF and IL-1β; UVA also induces a redox dependent release of MIF in keratinocytes, which, in turn, activates the production of active granzyme b. MIF-mediated granzyme b induction cause fibronectin degradation, and MIF also mediates the upregulation of MMP-1 (MMP-13), which ultimately leads to dermal collagen degradation.

Conclusion

It has now become evident that UV-radiation significantly stimulates the production of MIF in the skin. UV-induced MIF strongly mediates the enhancement of collagen degradation and basement membrane damage, which occurs primarily through the activation of MMP-9 and MMP-2 in the skin.

Furthermore, UV-induced IL-1β and MIF interrelated loops also induce MMP-1 and thus may contribute to the loss of interstitial collagen. Therefore, the identification of these new mechanisms will help us to understand the precise role of MIF in UV-induced dermal connective tissue damage, which ultimately leads to photoaging.

Acknowledgments

These experiments were carried out in collaboration with researchers whose work appears in the references.

References

[1] Matsumura, Y; Ananthaswamy HN. Short-term and long-term cellular and molecular events following UV irradiation of skin: implications for molecular medicine. *Expert Rev Mol Med.*, 2002, 4, 1-22.

[2] Tenkate, TD. Occupational exposure to ultraviolet radiation: a health risk assessment. *Rev Environ Health.*, 1999, 14, 187-209.

[3] Cho, HS; Kwak, DH; Choi, IS; Park, HK; Kang, SJ; Yoo, HS; Lee, MS; Oh, KW; Hong, JT. Inhibitory effect of! proanthocyanidin on ultraviolet B irradiation-inducedmelanogenesis. J. Toxicol. *Environ. Health A.*, 2009, 72, 1475-1483.

[4] F'guyer, S; Afaq, F; Mukhtar, H. Photochemoprevention of skin cancer by botanical agents. *Photodermatol.*, 2003, 19, 56-72.

[5] Lavker, RM. Structural alterations in exposed and unexposed aged skin. *J Invest Dermatol.*, 1979, 73, 559-566.

[6] Lavker, RM; Kligman, AM. Chronic heliodermatitis: a morphologic evaluation of chronic actinic dermal damage with emphasis on the role of mast cells. *J Invest Dermatol.*, 1988, 90, 325-330.

[7] Gilchrest, BA. Skin aging and photoaging: an overview. *J Am Acad Dermatol.*, 1989, 21, 610-613.

[8] Farkas, B; Magyarlaki, M; Csete, B; Nemeth, J; Rabloczky, G; Bernath, S; Literati Nagi, P; Sumegi, B. Reduction of acute photodamage in skin by topical application of a novel PARP inhibitor. *Biochem Pharmacol.*, 2002, 63, 921-932.

[9] Kulms, D; Zeise, E; Poppelmann, B; Schwarz, T. DNA damage, death receptor activation and reactive oxygen species contribute to ultraviolet radiation-induced apoptosis in an essential and independent pathway. *Oncogene.*, 2002, 21, 5844-5851.

[10] Kulms, D; Schwarz, T. Independent contribution of three different pathways to ultraviolet-B-induced apoptosis. *Biochem Pharmacol.*, 2002, 6, 837-841.

[11] Assefa, Z; Laethem, AV; Garmyn, M; Agostinis, P. Ultraviolet radiation-induced apoptosis in keratinocytes: on the role of cytosolic factors. *Biochim Biophys Acta.*, 2005, 1755, 90-106.

[12] Kondo, S. The roles of cytokines in photoaging. *J Dermatol Sci.*, 2000, 23, 30-36.

[13] Kupper, TS; Chua, AO; Flood, P; McGuire, J; Gubler, U. Interleukin 1 gene expression in cultured human keratinocytes is augmented by ultraviolet irradiation. *J. Clin. Invest.*, 1987, *80*, 430-436.

[14] Rutter, JL; Benbow, U; Coon, CI; Brinckerhoff, CE. Cell-type specific regulation of human interstitial collagenase-1 gene expression by interleukin-1 beta (IL-1 beta) in human fibroblasts and BC-8701 breast cancer cells. *J Cell Biochem.*, 1997, 66, 322-336.

[15] Kirnbauer, R; Köck, A; Neuner, P; Forster, E; Krutmann, J; Urbanski, A; Schauer, E; Ansel, JC; Schwarz, T; Luger, TA. Regulation of epidermal cell interleukin-6 production by UV light and corticosteroids. *J Invest Dermatol*, 1991, 96, 484-489.

[16] Köck, A; Schwarz, T; Kirnbauer, R; Urbanski, A; Perry, P; Ansel, JC; Luger, TA. Human keratinocytes are a source for tumor necrosis factor alpha: evidence for synthesis and release upon stimulation with endotoxin or ultraviolet light. *J Exp Med.*, 1990, 172, 1609-1614.

[17] Bashir, M.M; Sharma M.R; Werth, V.P. TNF-alpha production in the skin, *Arch.Dermatol Res.*, 2009, 301, 87-91.

[18] Dinarello, CA; Cannon, JG; Wolff, SM; Bernheim, HA; Beutler, B; Cerami, A; Figari, IS; Palladino, MA, Jr; O'Connor, JV. Tumor necrosis factor (cachectin) is an endogenous pyrogen and induces production of interleukin 1. *J. Exp. Med.*, 1986, 163, 1433-1450.

[19] Schwarz, A; Bhardwaj, R; Aragane, Y; Mahnke, K; Riemann, H; Metze, D; Luger, TA; Schwarz, T. Ultraviolet-B-induced apoptosis of keratinocytes: evidence for partial involvement of tumor necrosis factor-alpha in the formation of sunburn cells. *J. Invest. Dermatol.*, 1995, 104, 922-997.

[20] Yoshizumi, M; Nakamura, T; Kato, M; Ishioka, T; Kozawa, K; Wakamatsu, K; Kimura, H. Release of cytokines/chemokines and cell death in UVB-irradiated human keratinocytes, HaCaT, *Cell Biol. Int.*, 2008, 32, 1405-1411.

[21] Peus, D; Vasa, R.A; Meves, A; Pott, M; Beyerle, A; Squillace, K; Pittelkow, MR. H2O2 is an important mediator of UVB-induced EGF-receptor phosphorylation in cultured keratinocytes. *J Invest Dermatol.*, 1998, 110, 966-971.

[22] Bokov, A; Chaudhuri, A; Richardson, A. The role of oxidative damage and stress in aging. *Mech Ageing Dev.*, 2004, 125, 811-826.

[23] Halliwell, B. Antioxidant defence mechanisms: from the beginning to the end (of the beginning). *Free Radic Res.*, 1999, 31, 261–272.

[24] Fuchs, J; Huflejt, ME; Rothfuss, LM; Wilson, DS; Carcamo, G; Packer, L. Impairment of enzymic and nonenzymic antioxidants in skin by UVB irradiation. *J Invest Dermatol.*, 1989,93, 769-773.

[25] Kammeyar, A; Luiten, RM. Oxidation events and skin aging. *Ageing Res Rev.*, 2015, 21, 16-29.

[26] Scharffetter-Kochanek, K; Wlaschek, M; Brenneisen, P; Schauen, M; Blaudschun, R; Wenk, J. UV-Induced Reactive Oxygen Species in Photocarcinogenesis and Photoaging. *Biol Chem.*, 1997, 378, 1247-1257.

[27] Birkedal-Hansen, H. Catabolism and turnover of collagens: collagenases. *Methods Enzymol.*, 1987, 144, 140-171.

[28] Stricklin, GP; Hoidal, JR. Oxidant-mediated inactivation of TIMP. *Matrix Suppl.*, 1992, 1, 235.

[29] Masaki, H. Role of antioxidants in the skin: Anti-aging effects. *J Dermatol Sci.*, 2010, 58, 85-90.

[30] Afaq, H; Mukhtar, H. Botanical antioxidants in the preventation of photocarcinogenesis and photoaging. *Exp Dermatol.*, 2006, 15, 678-684.

[31] Yoshihisa, Y; Honda, A; Zhao, QL; Makino T; Abe, R; Matsui, K; Shimizu, H; Miyamoto, Y; Kondo, T; Shimizu, T. Protective effects of platinum nanoparticles against UV-induced epidermal inflammation. *Exp Dermatol.*, 2010, 19, 1000-1006.

[32] Bloom, BR; Bennett, B. Mechanism of a reaction *in vitro* associated with delayed-type hypersensitivity. *Science.*, 1966, 153, 80-82.

[33] David, JR. Delayed hypersensitivity *in vitro*: its mediation by cell-free substances formed by lymphoid cell-antigen interaction. *Proc Natl Acad Sci USA.*, 1966, 56, 72-77

[34] Weiser, WY; Temple, PA; Witek-Giannotti, JS., et al. Molecular cloning of a cDNA encoding a human macrophage migration inhibitory factor. *Proc Natl Acad Sci USA.*, 1989, 86, 7522-7526.

[35] Bernhagen, J; Calandra, T; Mitchell, RA; Martin, SB; Tracey, KJ; Voelter, W; Manogue, KR; Cerami, A; Bucala, R. MIF is a pituitary-derived cytokine that potentiates lethal endotoxaemia. *Nature.*, 1993, 365, 756-759.

[36] Calandra, T; Bernhagen, J; Mitchell, RA; Bucala R. The macrophage is an important and previously unrecognized source of macrophage migration inhibitory factor. *J Exp Med.*, 1994, 179, 1895-902.

[37] Nishihira, J. Macrophage Migration inhibitory factor (MIF): Its essential role in the immune system and cell growth. *J Interferon Cytokine Res.*, 2000, 20, 751-762.

[38] Meyer-Siegler, K; Hudson, PB. Enhanced expression of macrophage migration inhibitory factor in prostatic adenocarcinoma metastases. *Urology.*, 1996, 48, 448-452.

[39] Bando, H; Matsumoto, G; Bando, M; Muta, M; Ogawa, T; Funata, N; Nishihira, J; Koike, M; Toi, M. Expression of macrophage migration inhibitory factor in human breast cancer: association with nodal spread. *Jpn J Cancer Res.*, 2002, 93, 389-396.

[40] Shimizu, T; Abe, R; Nakamura, H; Ohkawara, A; Suzuki, M; Nishihira, J. High expression of macrophage migration inhibitory factor in human melanoma cells and its role in tumor cell growth and angiogenesis. *Biochem Biophys Res Commun.*, 1999, 264, 751-758.

[41] Chesney, J; Metz, C; Bacher, M; Peng, T; Meinhardt, A; Bucala, R. An essential role for macrophage migration inhibitory factor (MIF) in angiogenesis and the growth of a murine lymphoma. *Mol Med.*, 1999, 5,181-191.

[42] Calandra, T; Bernhagen, J; Metz, C.N; Spiegel, L.A; Bacher, M; Donnelly, T; Cerami, A; Bucala, R. MIF as a glucocorticoid-induced modulator of cytokine production. *Nature.*, 1995, 377, 68-71.

[43] Rosengren, E; Bucala, R; Aman, P; Jacobsson, L; Odh, G; Metz, CN; Rorsman, H. The immunoregulatory mediator macrophage migration

inhibitory factor (MIF) catalyzes a tautomerization reaction. *Mol. Med.*, 1996, *2*, 143-149.

[44] Roger, T; David, J; Glauser, MP; Calandra, T. MIF regulates innate immune responses through modulation of Toll-like receptor 4. *Nature.*, 2001, *414*, 920-924.

[45] Welford, S.M; Bedogni, B; Gradin, K; Poellinger, L; Broome Powell, M; Giaccia, A.J. HIF1alpha delays premature senescence through the activation of MIF. *Genes Dev.*, 2006, 20, 3366–3371.

[46] Wistow, GJ; Shaughnessy, MP; Lee, DC; Hodin, J; Zelenka, PS. A macrophage migration inhibitory factor is expressed in the differentiating cells of the eye lens. *Proc Natl Acad Sci USA.*, 1993, 90, 1272-1275.

[47] Nemajerova, A; Mena, P; Fingerle-Rowson, G; Moll, U.M; Petrenko, O. Impaired DNA damage checkpoint response in MIF-deficient mice. *EMBO J.*, 2007, 26, 987-997.

[48] Shimizu, T; Ohkawara, A; Nishihira, J; Sakamoto, W. Identification of macrophage migration inhibitory factor (MIF) in human skin and its immmunohistochemical localization. *FEBS Lett.*, 1996, 381, 199–202.

[49] Foote, A; Kipen, Y; Santos, L; Leech, M; Morand, EF. Macrophage migration inhibitory factor in systemic lupus erythematosus. *J Rheumatol.*, 2004, 31, 268-273.

[50] Fisher, GJ; Wang, ZQ; Datta, SC; Varani, J; Kang, S; Voorhees, JJ. Pathophysiology of premature skin aging induced by ultraviolet light. *N Engl J Med.*, 1997, 337, 1419-1428.

[51] Ohnishi, Y; Tajima, S; Akiyama, M; Ishibashi, A; Kobayashi, R; Horii, I. Expression of elastin-related proteins and matrix metalloproteinases in actinic elastosis of sun-damaged skin. *Arch Dermatol Res.*, 2000, 292, 27-31.

[52] Brenneisen, P; Oh, J; Wlaschek, M; Wenk, J; Briviba, K; Hommel, C; Herrmann, G; Sies, H; Scharffetter-Kochanek, K. Ultraviolet B wavelength dependence for the regulation of two major matrix-metalloproteinases and their inhibitor TIMP-1 in human dermal fibroblasts. *Photochem Photobiol.*, 1996, 64, 877-885.

[53] Zaid, MA; Afaq, F; Syed, DN; Dreher, M; Mukhtar, H. Inhibition of UVB-mediated oxidative stress and markers of photoaging in immortalized HaCaT keratinocytes by pomegranate polyphenol extract POMx. *Photochem.Photobiol.*, 2007, 83, 882-888.

[54] Chiang, HM; Chiu, HH; Liao, ST; Chen, YT; Chang, HC; Wen, KC. Isoflavonoid-rich flemingia macrophylla extract attenuates UVB-

induced skin damage by scavenging reactive oxygen species and inhibiting MAP kinase and MMP expression. *Evid. Based Complement. Altern. Med.*, 2013, 2013, 696879.

[55] Contet-Audonneau, JL; Jeanmaire, C; Pauly, G. A histological study of human wrinkle structures: comparison between sun-exposed areas of the face, with or without wrinkles, and sun-protected areas. *Br J Dermatol.*, 1999, 140, 1038-1047.

[56] Shimizu, T; Abe, R; Ohkawara, A; Nishihira, J. Ultraviolet B radiation up-regulates the production of macrophage migration inhibitory factor (MIF) in human epidermal keratinocytes. *J Invest Dermatol*, 1999, 112, 210-215.

[57] Watanabe, H; Shimizu, T; Nishihira, J; Abe, R; Nakayama, T; Taniguchi, M; Sabe, H; Ishibashi T; Shimizu, H. Ultraviolet A- induced production of matrix metalloproteinase-1 mediated by macrophage migration inhibitory factor (MIF) in human dermal fibroblasts. *J Biol Chem.*, 2004, 279, 1676-1683.

[58] Yoshihisa, Y; Norisugi, O; Matsunaga, K; Nishihira, J; Shimizu, T. Involvement of MIF in Basement Membrane Damage in Chronically UVB-Exposed Skin in Mice. *PLoS One.*, 2014, 9(2), e89569. doi:10.1371/journal.pone.0089569

[59] Honda, A; Abe, R; Makino, T; Norisugi, O; Fujita, Y; Watanabe, H; Nishihira, J; Iwakura, Y; Yamagishi, S; Shimizu, H; Shimizu, T. Interleukin-1b and macrophage migration inhibitory factor (MIF) in dermal fibroblasts mediate UVA-induced matrix metalloproteinase-1expression. *J Dermatol Sci.*, 2008, 49, 63-72.

[60] Hernandez-Pigeon, H; Jean, C; Charruyer, A; Haure, MJ; Baudouin, C; Charveron, M; Quillet-Mary, A; Laurent, G. UVA induces granzyme B in human keratinocytes through MIF: implication in extracellular matrix remodeling. *J Biol Chem.*, 2007, 282, 8157-8164.

Index

D

E

F

G

H

J

K

L

M

N

O

P

Q

R

S

T

U

V